My Birdsongs in Clinical Neurology

My Birdsongs in

Clinical Neurology

Sarosh M Katrak

Professor Emeritus
Department of Neurology
Grant Medical College and Sir JJ Group of Hospitals
Emeritus Director
Department of Neurology
Jaslok Hospital and Research Centre
Mumbai, Maharashtra, India

Foreword

Bhim Sen Singhal

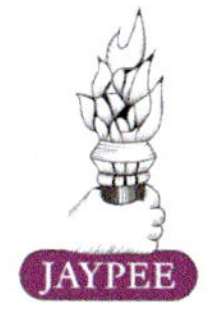

JAYPEE BROTHERS MEDICAL PUBLISHERS
The Health Sciences Publisher
New Delhi | London

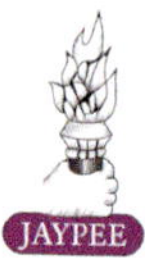

Jaypee Brothers Medical Publishers (P) Ltd

Headquarters
EMCA House
23/23-B, Ansari Road, Daryaganj
New Delhi 110 002, India
Landline: +91-11-23272143,
+91-11-23272703
+91-11-23282021, +91-11-23245672
E-mail: jaypee@jaypeebrothers.com

Corporate Office
Jaypee Brothers Medical Publishers (P) Ltd.
4838/24, Ansari Road, Daryaganj
New Delhi 110 002, India
Phone: +91-11-43574357
Fax: +91-11-43574314
E-mail: jaypee@jaypeebrothers.com

Overseas Office
JP Medical Ltd.
83, Victoria Street, London
SW1H 0HW (UK)
Phone: +44-20 3170 8910
E-mail: info@jpmedpub.com

EU GPSR Authorised Representative
Logos Europe, 9 rue Nicolas Poussin
17000, La Rochelle, France
Phone: +33 (0) 6 67 93 73 78
E-mail: Contact@logoseurope.eu

Website: www.jaypeebrothers.com
Website: www.jaypeedigital.com

Inquiries for bulk sales may be solicited at: jaypee@jaypeebrothers.com

***My Birdsongs in Clinical Neurology* / Sarosh M Katrak**

First Edition: 2024, Reprint: **2025**

ISBN: 978-93-5696-628-4

Printed in India

Dedications

This book is dedicated to:

My wife Ahalya. She has been my most severe critic and at the same time my most loyal supporter. Without her help and patience, this book would not have seen the light of day.
But, above all, for her eternal love.

My children, Shehzad and Gitanjali, for their continued love and affection and also for their understanding at a very tender age. They sacrificed many a days of their childhood so that I could pursue my career in neurology.

My mentors Professor Noshir H Wadia and Professor Bhim Sen Singhal in Mumbai, India, and Professor Martin Pollock in Dunedin, New Zealand. I learnt clinical neurology from their "birdsongs" and I am what I am today because of them.

My students who kept me up to date by their questions and also their enthusiasm for neurology.

Lastly, to all my patients, who gave freely of themselves so that I could learn the practice of neurology and improve myself.

Foreword

I consider it a great honor to have been asked to write the foreword for the book *"My Birdsongs in Clinical Neurology"* by Professor Sarosh M Katrak. Initially, I was intrigued by the title of this book, particularly the word "Birdsongs". In the preface, he has given the explanation why he used the word "Birdsongs". After reading it, I feel that the title is appropriate for a book on clinical methods, particularly the word "Birdsongs".

Professor Katrak is well known for his teaching skills with emphasis on clinical examination. He is also passionate about his hobbies of photography and calligraphy. From his keen sense of observation, he has introduced new clinical signs such as the "hair loss" sign, suggestive of diabetic distal sensory peripheral neuropathy, the "*namaste*" and "worn out heel" signs for detecting subtle hemiatrophy, and the "Parvati" sign, an observation he made while visiting the Ellora caves. Because of his passion for calligraphy, he observed that the inscriptions at the entrance of the Taj Mahal had adopted the principles of acuity of vision long before Snellen reported it in his famous chart. He has laid great emphasis on the art of history taking and drawing conclusions from it before proceeding to examination and investigation.

In the following chapters, Professor Katrak has dealt with the anatomy and relevant physiology of the nervous system. He explained the higher cortical dysfunctions correlating with the parts of brain involved, anatomy of cranial nerves, spinal cord, and related functions. He has also mentioned the common illnesses encountered and given the tips for quick and appropriate diagnosis. He has simplified the complex dysfunction and management of the urinary bladder. In the last chapter, he has given very useful tips for the practicing neurologists.

I thoroughly enjoyed reading this book. I have learnt a few lessons which I will make use of when seeing my patients. I strongly recommend this book not only for postgraduate students in medicine and neurology but also for practicing neurologists.

Bhim Sen Singhal
MD DSc(Honorary) FRCP FAMS
Director
Department of Neurology
Bombay Hospital Institute of Medical Sciences
Mumbai, Maharashtra, India

Preface

If one is an avid bird watcher, one realizes that some of the species of birds are dwindling. There are many reasons for these dwindling numbers. One of the main reasons is that man is encroaching on their environment through development. As a direct consequence of that, the adult male birds have to fly further and further to get food for their young ones. A direct result of this is that the adult males are unable to teach their young ones the male birdsongs, which are an essential part of mating and procreation.

In a similar vein, I feel that advances in the field of neuroimaging have encroached upon the environment of clinical neurology. Thus, the art of clinical neurology is being taught less and less. After over 50 years of teaching experience, I thought that I would pen some of my experiences in clinical neurology—"My Birdsongs"—for the benefit of postgraduates and young neurologists. The purpose of this small book is not to replace a thorough and standardized textbook of neurological examination but to complement it. It contains suggestions on how to elicit a history in appropriate depth as well as clinical tips which make the neurological examination easier without losing its accuracy.

I begin with some observations I have made over the years in clinical practice. We have published one of these—the "hair loss sign"—but in the Indian Journal of Endocrinology and Metabolism where it did not get much attention of the neurologists. I have not published the other three but would like to document them in this book. Firstly, the combined "*namaste*" and "worn out heel" sign is useful in arriving at a diagnosis of hemiatrophy with or without hemiplegia and epilepsy. The second—Herman Snellen versus Amanat Khan—is a result of my passion for calligraphy and the third—the "Parvati" sign—is rather peculiar to India and resulted from my passion for photography. The rest of the chapters deal with some clinical aspects of higher mental functions, the 12 cranial nerves, some aspects of the motor and sensory systems, and the physiological basis of tone and deep tendon reflexes. Chapter 15 reflects my bias for neurocritical care. On the other hand, the neurogenic bladder has always been a confusing and difficult topic for me to grasp. Chapter 16 is my attempt at simplifying this complex topic. In the last chapter, I have given explanations for some of the statements I have made to emphasize a clinical point.

As mentioned earlier, this monogram is by no means complete. I undertook this project to show subtle ways to make a detailed neurological examination easy and enjoyable and how to interpret the data elicited from the history and an accurate clinical examination, to achieve a provisional diagnosis using clinical reasoning. I hope you enjoy reading "My Birdsongs" as much as I enjoyed writing them, literally, for the future generation of clinical neurologists.

Sarosh M Katrak

Acknowledgments

This book would have never been literally written were it not for the encouragement I received from my core family, close friends, and associates. I am indebted to all of them. I extend my sincere thanks to Professor Bhim Sen Singhal, who graciously consented to write the foreword for this book but only after reading the entire manuscript. I am also grateful to my wife, Ahalya, not only for typing and proofreading the manuscript but also for helping me immensely with many of the figures. The willing help given by Dr Arjun G Shah in typing the latter half of the manuscript is also duly acknowledged. My sincere thanks to Mr Ravisankar Viswanathan, Cluster Head – CNS, Sun Pharma for obtaining near impossible articles for me. Finally, my sincere thanks to the management of Jaypee Brothers Medical Publishers at New Delhi and Mumbai, India, for publishing this book, and particularly Ms Kritika Dua (Senior Commissioning Editor), Mr Ashish Kumar (Business Manager), and Mr Naman Singh (Development Editor) for their assistance, cooperation, and support throughout the publication of this book.

Sarosh M Katrak

Contents

CHAPTER 1

My Observations Over the Years

OBSERVATION 1: THE HAIR LOSS SIGN

My interest in peripheral neuropathies is well known since I published my work on gold neuropathy in 1980. While examining patients with diabetic sensory neuropathy, I observed loss of hair distally in the lower limbs in a stocking distribution and that it coincided with the distal sensory loss. With subsequent experience, this led me to the presence of a peripheral neuropathy just by observing the hair loss **(Figs. 1.1A and B)**.

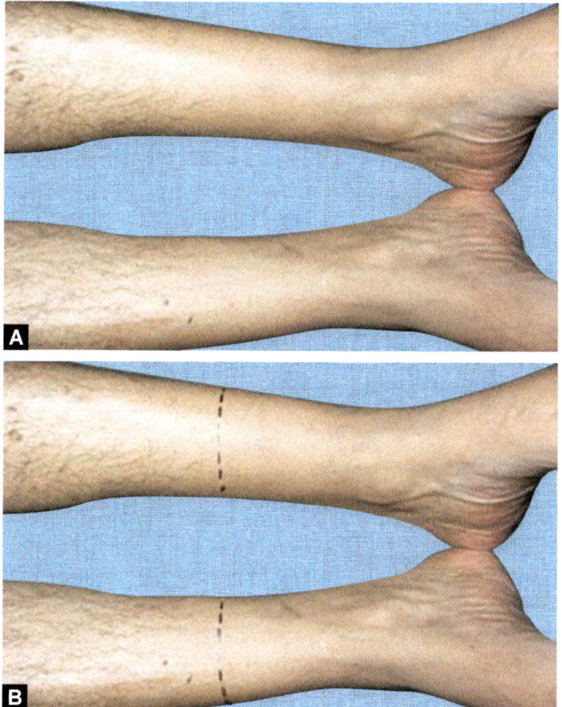

FIGS. 1.1A AND B: Hair loss sign.

Dr Satish Khadilkar put two of his students, Dr Amit Choudhary and Dr Riddhi Patel, to test the veracity of this observation. We studied 107 patients with a mean age of 69.1 years and a mean duration of diabetes for 8.7 years. The conclusion from the study was "hair loss sign, when present, can be used as a rapid and reliable clinical indicator of moderate to severe neuropathy". This would also include, in my opinion, that there is an element of autonomic neuropathy because, I believe that the hair loss is due to autonomic denervation of the hair follicle. The limitations of this study were that there was no hair loss in early and mild neuropathy and in fashionable ladies, depilation vitiated this sign. We published our findings in a letter to the Editor of the Indian Journal of Endocrinology and Metabolism in 2019. Dr Khadilkar, who was the corresponding author, noted a good response from physicians and endocrinologists but a lukewarm response from neurologists. That is the reason for including this observation in this monogram. We were very happy when Dr Khadilkar received a letter from a physician from a teaching hospital in the United Kingdom which stated "*...please could I have permission to use the photo for teaching? We will print the photos and show it to about 40 students in a practice examination...*" This showed that the hair loss sign was accepted.

OBSERVATION 2: THE NAMASTE AND WORN-OUT HEEL SIGN

One of the causes of focal epilepsy in childhood and young adults is the hemiplegia, hemiatrophy, and epilepsy syndrome (HHE). When the hemiplegia and hemiatrophy are obvious, the diagnosis is also obvious. When the hemiatrophy is subtle, without any weakness, the clinical diagnosis is more difficult, particularly if there is no history of convulsions. Let me illustrate this point with a case vignette.

SJ, male, 37 years, was diagnosed with type 2 diabetes mellitus (T2DM). He was advised oral hypoglycemic agents (OHAs) together with a strict diet. However, he discontinued his medication after 15 days. In September 2021, he noticed asymptomatic thinning of his left thigh. In May 2023, he complained of severe burning pain radiating along the anterior and medial aspects of the left thigh. This was associated with difficulty in walking as his left knee would buckle under his weight. The pain was more in the sitting posture and a shade less in the supine position. There was a history suggestive of fasciculations in the left thigh. His physician made a provisional diagnosis of diabetic amyotrophy and advised strict dietary control and OHAs. In the last 3 months, he lost 6 kg body weight, which he attributed to the strict diet. On examination, there was wasting predominantly in the left thigh. The left quadriceps was distinctly weaker compared to the right, the left knee jerk was absent, and there was L2-3-4 hypoesthesia. All the other deep tendon reflexes were brisker than those on the right. The plantar response was flexor on the right and equivocal on the left.

The differential diagnosis was between diabetic amyotrophy and lumbar plexopathy. The only question was to explain the wasted left thigh of nearly 2 years' duration and the soft pyramidal signs on the left side. This suggested that on a background of a "grumbling problem," he had an acute flare-up in May 2023. My clinical reasoning was that the patient had noticed the wasting in September 2021 and that it was an old problem of hemiatrophy.

Measuring the length of the upper and lower limbs from fixed symmetrical bony points is a time consuming and tedious task. What I do is to ask the patient to put both his/her elbows on my desk, join the forearms side by side and perpendicular to the surface of my desk, and do a "*Namaste*". You then see whether the tips of the fingers are at the same level. This maneuver is easy and establishes the diagnosis of hemiatrophy by detecting the asymmetry in the length of the forearm and hand. This is what I call the "*Namaste*" sign **(Figs. 1.2A and B)**.

If there is a subtle hemiatrophy involving the lower limbs (as it was, in this case), one can compare the length of the two feet placed side by side **(Fig. 1.3A)**. In this case, there was a distinct difference, which had gone unnoticed throughout his life. Another easy way to establish this is to look at the heels of the patient's *chappals* or shoes. Because the normal lower limb is longer, the heel on that side is more worn out as it scrapes the ground much more—the "*worn-out heel*" sign **(Fig. 1.3B)**.

Secondly, the shoe on the hemiatrophic side is more creased. Lastly, ask the patient, when he goes to buy a new pair of footwear, which side does he try on. It will invariably be the normal side. Thus, the "*Namaste*" and "*worn-out heel*" signs are an easy way to help you to establish a subtle long-standing hemiatrophy and could help you in establishing a diagnosis of hemiatrophy with or without hemiparesis or focal epilepsy.

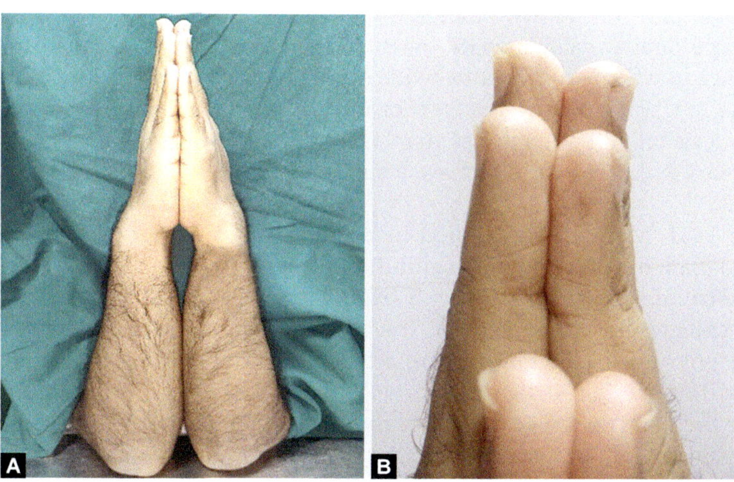

FIGS. 1.2A AND B: (A) *Namaste* sign; (B) Close-up of the same patient showing an asymmetry in the length of the fingers.

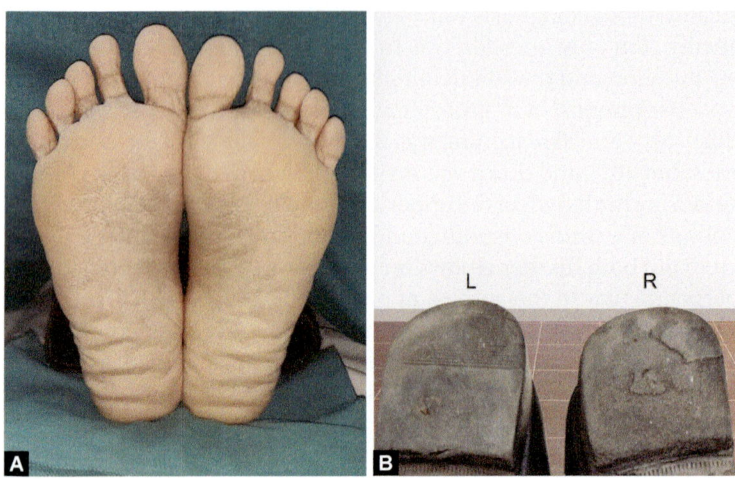

FIGS. 1.3A AND B: (A) Asymmetry of the feet; (B) Worn-out heel sign.

OBSERVATION 3: SNELLEN VERSUS AMANAT KHAN

Those of us who wear spectacles are familiar with Snellen's chart which is used to test our acuity of vision (A/V) and the degree of refractory error. This chart was scientifically developed by the Dutch ophthalmologist Herman Snellen in 1862 and is still the global standard for refractory error after over 160 years. The most significant innovation was his use of especially designed characters which he called "optotypes". Standard or normal vision was measured as the ability to read the line of optotype when they subtend an angle of 5° to the eye—thus the greater the distance, the larger is the optotype. Snellen calculated the height of each optotype line to represent the distance at which an individual with normal vision can read the optotype. As the A/V was measured at 20 ft or 6 m, 20/20 or 6/6 was considered as normal vision. Although this principle was scientifically established in 1862, 230 years earlier, we in India have a superb example of this in Agra, the Taj Mahal.

In 1631, Mumtaz Mahal died in childbirth and the grieving emperor, Shah Jahan, decided to build a grand mausoleum in her memory. The task of adorning the mausoleum with exquisite calligraphy was given to the royal calligrapher Amanat Khan. The black border on the edges of the arch at the entrance of the mausoleum are actually Arabic calligraphy quoting verses from the Quran. If one looks at the calligraphy at eye level, at the base of the arch, and again at the top of the arch which is approximately 150 ft high, the size of the inscription looks exactly the same **(Fig. 1.4)**. If this is not a practical application of Snellen's principle of A/V, then what is? Kindly remember that this was done 230 years before Snellen's article.

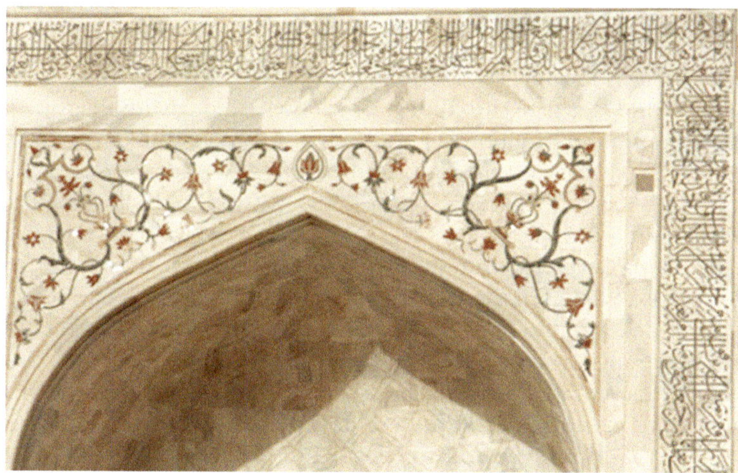

FIG. 1.4: Calligraphy on the arch of the Taj Mahal. The lower end of the vertical part is at approximately 100 ft and the horizontal part at 150 ft.

A word about Amanat Khan would be in order. His real name was Abd-al-Haq and he migrated from Shiraz in Iran in 1608 CE. Being a gifted calligrapher, Shah Jahan gave him the charge of the imperial library. On completion of the Taj Mahal, the emperor was so pleased with his work that he bestowed the title of Amanat Khan on him (Amanat means heirloom). He is credited with the creation of one of the five schools of Arabic calligraphy, Thuluth. This word in Arabic means one-third and if you look closely, one-third of each word slopes downward **(Fig. 1.5)**.

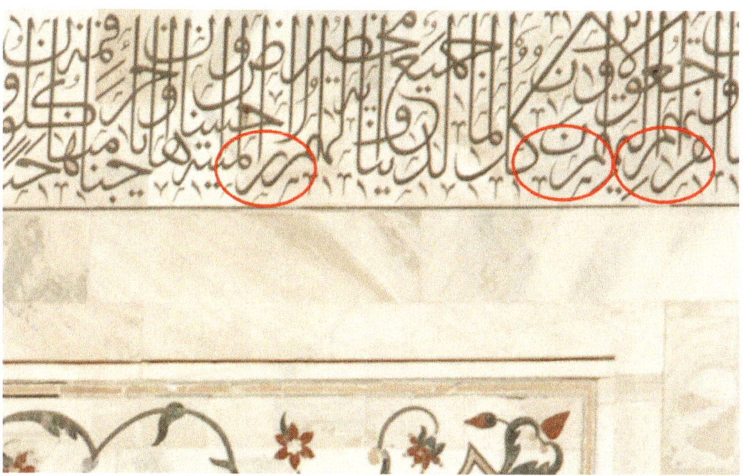

FIG. 1.5: Calligraphy on the Taj Mahal. Note the latter one-third of the letters slope downward. Details are given in the text.

OBSERVATION 4: THE PARVATI SIGN

The Ellora Caves located in the Aurangabad district of Maharashtra are an UNESCO World Heritage site. Today, Ellora caves, along with nearby Ajanta Caves, are protected monuments under the Archaeological Survey of India (ASI). The Ellora caves were excavated in three periods: An early Hindu period (~550–600 CE), a Buddhist phase (~600–730 CE), and a later Hindu and Jain phase (~730–950 CE).

In the Ellora Caves, cave number 16 features the largest monolithic (single piece) rock excavation in the world—The Kailash Temple, a chariot-shaped monument dedicated to Lord Shiva. It is a free-standing, multilevel temple complex covering an area twice the size of the Parthenon in Athens, Greece. The monolithic rock excavation, unlike other structures, began at the top and was done in the early Hindu period. It was estimated that the artisans removed 3 million cubic feet of stone weighing approximately 200,000 tons to carve out this temple complex. The Kailash Temple is a "wonder of the world" among rock-cut monuments and is considered a highly notable example of a temple construction from the first millennium of Indian history. It features sculptures depicting Hindu gods and goddesses as well as relief panels summarizing the two major Hindu epics.

One of the themes in the Kailash temple is the mural depicting the wedding of Lord Shiva to Parvati–Shiv vivah **(Fig. 1.6A)**. According to mythology, Lord Shiva eloped with Parvati in order to marry her. They went to Mount Kailash where Lord Brahma was to conduct the wedding rites along with Lord Vishnu. Again, according to mythology, Parvati's parents were in hot pursuit. Lord Shiva was in a hurry to finish the "*saat pheras*" around the holy fire. While performing the "*kanya daan*" traditionally, the bride places her right hand into the hand of the bridegroom. As Lord Shiva was in a great hurry, he placed his right hand into the hand of Parvati **(Fig. 1.6B)**, to her great embarrassment **(Fig. 1.6C)**. In the mural, this embarrassment is depicted by the position of Parvati's left big toe **(Fig. 1.6C, green arrow)** trying to grip her right big toe **(Fig. 1.6C, red arrow)**.

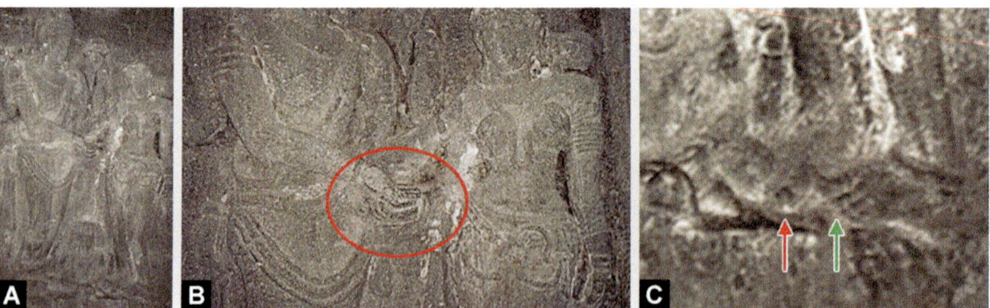

FIGS. 1.6A TO C: *Shiv vivah*. (A) Mural; (B) Hands; (C) Parvati's feet.
Courtesy: SMK.

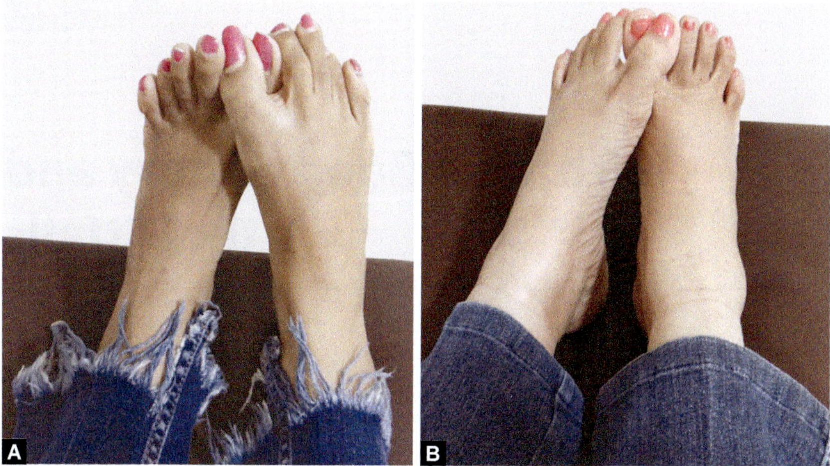

FIGS. 1.7A AND B: Two patients showing the "Parvati" sign.

When the ASI guide explained this to me, my thoughts went to many of my female patients. When I try to lift their *sari* or *churidar* above the ankle level in order to elicit the ankle jerk, they perform the same gesture of embarrassment as was depicted in the mural. This is what I call the "Parvati" sign **(Figs. 1.7A and B)**.

It is seen more frequently in women hailing from rural and semiurban regions. In the urban areas, it occurs with a greater frequency in orthodox individuals; nevertheless, I have also seen it in modern women **(Figs. 1.7A and B)**. It transcends religion and cultural habits, but it is typically Indian! In the 2 years of my stay in New Zealand, I do not recall seeing the "Parvati" sign in a single female patient. What amazes me is that the artisans in ancient India depicted this characteristic gesture of embarrassment of an Indian woman over 1,600 years ago and how it has persisted through the centuries.

RECOMMENDED ARTICLES

1. Katrak S, Choudhary A, Patel R, Khadilkar S. A simple and reliable clinical indicator for rapid evaluation of neuropathy in busy diabetic clinics: "Hair loss sign." Indian J Endocrin Metabol. 2019;23(5):585-6.
2. Kochhar A. Sarai Amanat Khan: Legacy of the Taj calligrapher. Live History, India, July 10, 2019.
3. Snellen H. Probebuchstaber zur Bestimmang der Schscharfe. Utrecht: Van de Weijer; 1862.

CHAPTER 2

Eliciting a Good History and the Pitfalls

Certain ground rules are necessary in eliciting a good history.

1. Always put the date/time before documenting your history. Also write case seen by Dr ... and designation.
2. Avoid terms like "7 days ago, the patient experienced ..." If the history was taken on July 25, 2023, instead of 7 days ago, put on "18th July the patient experienced ..." Mentioning specific dates establishes an exact chronological time frame to the history.
3. If a specific date is not forthcoming, write end of July or fourth week of July.
4. At the end of the history and findings, put your clinical reasoning together with the provisional diagnosis. Make your mistakes and correct them when the patient is seen by the consultant. This way, you will improve your clinical reasoning faster. I often say *"if you don't make mistakes, you will never learn"*.

The great medical philosopher Sir William Osler once said, *"the good physician treats the disease, the great physician treats the patient who has the disease".*

A great physician differs from a good physician because he understands the patient's entire story and takes a holistic view of the patient. He understands the patient's disease, their new problems, their social situation, and their beliefs and fears. How can you achieve all this? One has to develop excellent communication skills and take a history in appropriate depth. The next step is to perform a targeted physical examination based on the clues obtained from the history. Thus, eliciting a good neurological history is an art in which the patient will give you two important aspects of the diagnosis–where is the lesion and what is the lesion.

"You have two eyes and two ears and only one mouth: therefore you must see and hear twice as much as you speak". An old Chinese saying.

The above saying is really the secret to elicit a good neurological history. You have every opportunity to observe the patient (two eyes) and analyze the speech (two ears) while he/she is reciting the history. Also, note the posture and gait as he/she enters your consulting room. Do not interrupt the patient or caregiver in mid-sentence but ask your point when they have completed the history of that particular symptom. In young children, pay particular attention to what the mother is saying. I have often heard mothers say, "Doctor, I can look at her and know she is going to get a fit". Do not laugh at her because she is invariably right. While dealing with a patient of minimal cognitive impairment (MCI) or dementia, pay close attention to the history by the caregiver. An example from one of my patients illustrates this point. His wife had moderate-to-severe Alzheimer's disease (AD). He asked me, "Doctor, can't you do something for me? She does not give me a minute to myself. If I am having a bath, she is outside the door, saying come out soon, come out soon. She has practically become my shadow". I had to explain to him that patients with AD become so dependent on the caregiver that they constantly shadow them, exactly what he told me in the history.

In a case of ataxia, a dysarthric speech quickly separates cerebellar ataxia from sensory ataxia. If the patient has low-grade fever and diabetes, in India, always remember that "in the shadow of diabetes is tuberculosis". If in a case of young-onset epilepsy, you are suspecting neurocysticercosis, remember to ask the patient, "while having a bath and applying the soap, do you feel any lumps or bumps?". If the answer is yes, the patient may point to a subcutaneous cysticercus cyst, confirming your suspicion. Another patient's wife kept complaining that he keeps fiddling with the color adjustment of our TV. It did not take me long to establish that he had a defect of color vision.

At times, the patient literally gives you the diagnosis if you have knowledge of the condition. Again, I would like to illustrate this point by giving you examples from my experiences over the years:

- *The Jesuit priest who gave me his diagnosis*: This elderly Jesuit priest, originally from Italy, used to write letters to his family in Rome. His main complaint was that when he wrote letters, he had to lock himself up in his room. If he was disturbed or interrupted, "he could not read what he had written". This was in 1975 when writing letters was the main mode of communication. This priest had the disconnection syndrome of alexia without agraphia and literally gave me the diagnosis when he said, "I cannot read what I have written". He had a right homonymous hemianopia. Thus, all the visual information fell on the right visual cortex and there was no transfer of information to the left side because of a concurrent lesion in the splenium of the corpus callosum, thus the alexia (the curved arrow in **Fig. 2.1**). He could write because his Wernicke's area, angular gyrus, and motor area were intact–no agraphia. This was due to a glioma in the left parieto-occipital area, and unfortunately, he progressed further to alexia with agraphia and ultimately perished from his disease.
- The husband of another patient said, "she keeps bumping into objects on the left hand side. Look at her left shoulder, it is bruised! She also forgets recent things". His wife had a left temporal field of vision defect and

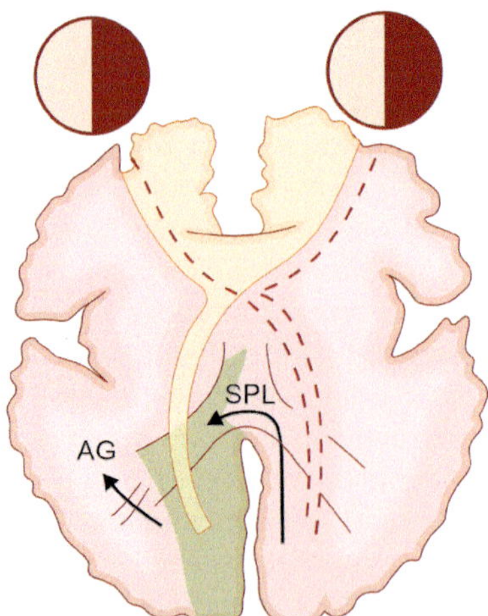

FIG. 2.1: Alexia without agraphia. Green area indicates area of the lesion. Explanation is given in the text.
(AG: angular gyrus; SPL: splenium of corpus callosum)

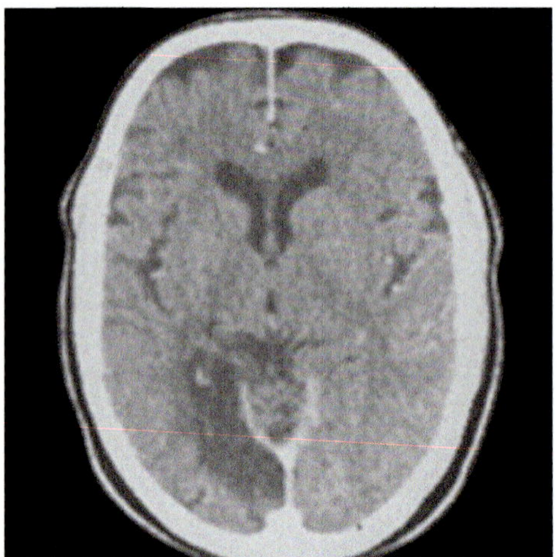

FIG. 2.2: Postcontrast CT scan showing right PCA infarct.
(CT: computed tomography; PCA: posterior cerebral artery)

together with the memory loss, it was easy to make a diagnosis of a right posterior cerebral artery infarct **(Fig. 2.2)**.

- This case emphasizes how close a differential diagnosis lies between syncope and epilepsy and how a detailed history resolves the issue. A 60-year-old male patient presented with a history of unexplained falls, which was diagnosed as epilepsy in a peripheral hospital. A detailed history also revealed that he was unable to relax his grip. A diagnosis of myotonic dystrophy was made and the falls were due to cardiac conduction tissue involvement in myotonic dystrophy.

- I was once called to see a 40-year-old female patient with an acute onset of right hemiplegia with an inability to speak. On examination, she had an upper motor neuron facial palsy with grade 0 power in the right upper and lower limbs together with a dense sensory loss to pain on the right-hand side. However, the tone and deep tendon reflexes (DTR) were normal and the right plantar response was flexor. I suspected a functional hemiplegia but was intrigued as to how a lay person had knowledge of a so-called upper motor neuron facial palsy with the hemiplegia. Digging further into the history, it transpired that she was the sole person in a large joint family who was given the responsibility of looking after her father-in-law who had a genuine right-sided stroke with aphasia. She was observant enough to notice that the lower facial weakness went with the hemiplegia. I felt that she deserved "her rest and attention". She was admitted into a hospital under my care and with suggestion therapy made a complete recovery.
- A 45-year-old male patient gave a history of insidious and progressive distal weakness, initially of the lower and then the upper limbs. Clinically, he had all the features of a distal symmetrical sensorimotor axonal neuropathy of uncertain etiology. As I was leaving his bedside at the JJ Hospital after examining him, he called me back and said, "Doctor sahib, I had this tattoo of my name 'Krishna' on my left forearm. Now I can hardly see it". I confirmed that the tattoo could be seen faintly and it gave me the diagnosis. Arsenic poisoning not only produces a sensorimotor axonal neuropathy but also increases the pigmentation of the skin. Blood and hair samples confirmed the diagnosis. How was he getting the arsenic? That is another story altogether, beyond the scope of this book, but a detailed history revealed the source of arsenic.
- A Sikh gentleman was admitted into another hospital under a rheumatologist because he had progressive history of joint pains, cerebellar ataxia, and peripheral neuropathy. No diagnosis was achieved, and he came under my care at the Jaslok Hospital. The most impressive finding was that this patient had severe alopecia with hair all over his pillowcase. On inquiring about it, his wife brought out a big bag full of his hair and stated that the alopecia started with his illness. It was thus very easy to make a diagnosis of thallium poisoning which was confirmed by blood, urine, and hair analysis.

Thallium is used in the production of fluorescent tube lights. The culprit had imported thallium on this excuse. Another interesting aspect of this case was the fact that the culprit had seen an episode on National Geographic in which there was an accidental contamination of water with thallium and the same water was used in the production of a cola which masked the taste of thallium. The patient was given thallium in a cola by the culprit who owed the patient large sums of money.

PITFALLS IN ELICITING A FAMILY HISTORY

Lastly, I would like to stress a few pitfalls in eliciting a family history in India. Let me begin with an example. The year was 1970 and I was a house-officer in the department of neurology under Dr NH Wadia (NHW). A 22-year-old Sikh gentleman with huge pseudohypertrophy of the calves and proximal hip girdle weakness was admitted in the ward. My co-house officer (HO) took the history and asked the patient if anybody in his family had a similar problem. "No!" was the prompt answer. The next morning, NHW came on the rounds and asked my co-HO about the family history and was surprised with a negative answer. NHW just nodded and asked the patient, "how many maternal uncles (mamas) do you have?" Three was the answer. NHW asked, "how many of them had calves like yours". The patient promptly replied that two of his uncles had such calves. Subsequently, my co-HO was very angry with the patient and asked why he gave NHW a positive family history. Promptly came the patient's answer, "you asked me if anybody in my family had a similar problem. My family is from my father's side and nobody has a similar problem". Moral of the story: In India, many communities consider the father's side as their family. In X-linked disorders, please inquire about the maternal side of the family, just as NHW did from his vast experience.

Another example is a family of facioscapulohumeral myopathy. As a registrar (1972), I asked the patient whether anybody in his family had a similar problem. The patient replied, "No, doctor. In fact, my younger brother is in the army". So I wrote, family history negative. One day, an army officer came to see the patient and I asked him if he was the patient's brother. When he said yes, I made a request to examine him. He also had facioscapulohumeral weakness. Hence, I inquired which branch of the army he was in. I was surprised that he was in the Signal Corp and in those days all he had to do was Morse code and wireless verbal messages. He had bilateral facial weakness and could not close his eyes completely. I got an inspiration and asked him, "how many family members sleep with their eyes half-closed?". "Almost all, that is our family trait". Moral of the lesson: When you suspect a familial problem, try and examine as many family members as possible and ask for simple activities of daily living which the weak muscles are supposed to do. For example, how many family members have difficulty in getting up from the Indian-style toilet when there is a history of hip-girdle weakness.

Lastly, a young girl with clinical and electrophysiological evidence of hereditary motor-sensory neuropathy came to me for an opinion. All I asked was, "how many family members have funny toes?" The mother promptly took off her shoes and showed me her hammer toes.

The other problem with family history in India is the blame or guilt complex. In X-linked disorders, particularly Duchenne's muscular dystrophy, I have known mothers to feel guilty and depressed. Good counseling is required in such cases together with an understanding spouse. Very often, an autosomal dominant disorder is hidden when matrimonial arrangements are made. If the problem is inherited from the paternal side, the matter is often accepted, but the blame game begins in a major form if the inheritance is from the maternal side. As I said earlier, the neurologist must tread carefully and counsel the family carefully seeking the help of a clinical psychologist if necessary.

RECOMMENDED ARTICLE

1. Centor RM. To be a Great Physician You Must Understand the Whole Story. MedGenMed. 2007;9(1):59.

CHAPTER 3

Higher Mental Functions

INTRODUCTION

A complete assessment of higher mental functions pertinent to each of the four lobes: frontal, parietal, temporal and occipital—is beyond the scope of this book. In this chapter I am only going to discuss a simplified assessment of aphasias and frontal lobe release reflexes.

SIMPLIFIED ASSESSMENT OF APHASIAS

Language is the ability to communicate through common symbols (alphabets) and is the most human attribute separating us from other species. Language develops during our childhood, initially through sound, touch, and color. Later, it develops through babbling, words, sentences, and then reading and writing. During this evolution, the individual also develops concepts about self and the environment; for example, to a child, C-A-T means a four-legged animal which says "meow", but to a medical student it may also mean computerized axial tomography. To a child, a mouse is a rodent but to a computer geek it is a tool.

Aphasia is the study of language disorders and should be distinguished from disorders of phonation, i.e., speech disorders. The main language circuit lies in the dominant hemisphere and is diagrammatically shown in **Figure 3.1**.

For hearing and answering, the sound waves are converted to electrical activity and reach Heschl's gyrus (superior temporal gyrus). Wernicke's area (left posterior temporal gyrus) lies next to the cortical area of hearing and is involved in the recognition and decoding of the patterns of spoken or written language. Here, there is an interaction between Wernicke's area and the angular gyrus (the area of concepts). This adds concepts from previous experiences to the decoded sounds and is converted into "electrical activity". This electrical activity is conveyed via Wernicke's loop to Broca's area (left anterior frontal gyrus). Broca's area contains "rules" by which spoken/ written language could be coded into an articulatory or a written form. These

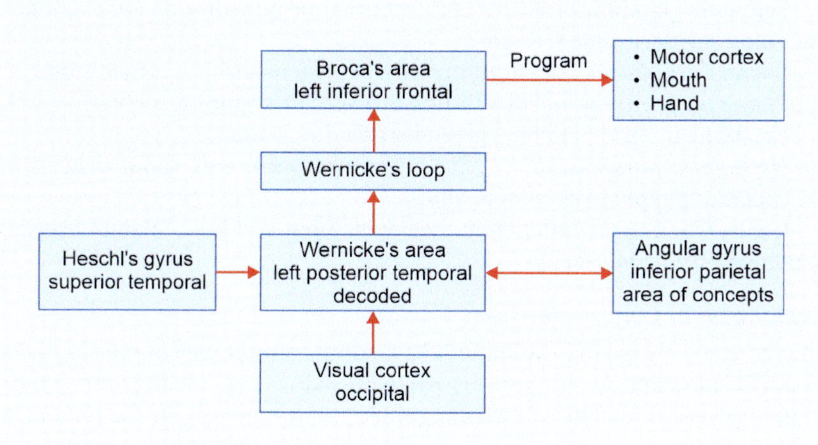

FIG. 3.1: Main language circuit in the dominant hemisphere.

programmed codes of the spoken/written answer are conveyed to the motor cortex of the larynx, mouth, and tongue for a verbal answer or the hand area for a written answer.

The circuit for reading and answering differs from the above only in the initial stages. The visual impulses fall on the visual cortex (occipital lobe) from where they are transmitted to Wernicke's area. The subsequent circuit and decoding are the same.

Evaluation of Aphasias

The bedside evaluation of aphasias are as follows:

- Spontaneous speech
- Comprehension of spoken speech
- Repetition
- Naming
- Reading: Aloud and for comprehension
- Writing: Copying written text, writing to dictation, and spontaneous sentences (comprehension)

Evaluation of Spontaneous Speech

This is easily done while eliciting the history or asking the patient to describe the nature of his work. In lesions, anterior to the sylvian fissure, the spontaneous speech is nonfluent and in posteriorly placed lesions it is fluent. During evaluation of spontaneous speech, one must note for prosody and semantic paraphasia.

Prosody is the rhythm of spoken speech and is described as melodic or nonmelodic.

Semantic paraphasia is the incorrect use or substitution of a similar-sounding word within a sentence.

- *Literal paraphasia*: Substitution of an incorrect word, e.g., grass is blue
- *Phonemic paraphasia*: Substitution of a similar-sounding incorrect word, e.g., bone instead of phone, gleen for green
- *Neologistic paraphasia*: A "new" incorrect word, e.g., spoot instead of spoon or peaper instead of people

Lastly, when the spontaneous speech is fluent and full of paraphasias, it becomes jargon aphasia.

Evaluation of Comprehension

This is tested by asking the patient to perform simple or complex activity to a spoken order. Avoid gestures while speaking, e.g., raising your hands in the upward direction when asking the patient to get up. If the patient is unable to do so, ask him to answer yes/no to simple questions or to point to a named object in the room.

Comprehension is rarely an all or none phenomenon. Initially, ask the patient to perform complex activity (a three-step command). If they are unable to do so, ask them to perform a simple activity or give yes/no answers when pointing to objects in the room. This is based on the severity of the comprehension dysfunction. Please note that bilateral body parts are easier to identify. Similarly, activities involving bilateral body parts are easier to perform.

Evaluation of Repetition

Ask the patient to repeat digits or common words: 9-8-7, five digits from your mobile number, or objects like house, pen, table, or chair. If he performs that, ask him to repeat a complex sentence. Lastly, try multisyllabic words like "no ifs, ands, or buts".

A tendency to repeat everything without comprehension is called echolalia. A predominantly repetition defect is seen in conduction aphasia (CA).

Evaluation of Naming

Assess the patient's response by confronting him with objects, body parts, or colors. He may be asked to name objects placed in his hands with his eyes closed (tactile stimulus) or by jingling a bunch of keys or a bell (auditory stimulus).

Defects of naming are not specific for aphasia. They can occur in nonaphasic disorders like acute confusional states or advanced dementia.

Evaluation of Reading

Reading is tested by asking the patient to read aloud without comprehension (like a parrot) and/or to read with understanding. The latter is done by asking the patient to interpret a complex sentence or failing which ask the patient to read aloud a written word and point to the object in the room.

Disorders of reading are developmental dyslexias in children (mild) to complete inability to read—alexias—in adults.

Evaluation of Writing

The patient may be asked to copy a written sentence, write a sentence to dictation, or write a few sentences about his work or daily routine. Copying is easier than writing to dictation and will be performed even when comprehension is mildly affected. On the other hand, writing spontaneous sentences involves intact comprehension. Therefore, this method of testing is in a descending extent of disability.

Classification of Aphasias

A few ground rules should be mentioned here before classifying aphasia which are as follows:

- *Aphasias are symptom complex; they are rarely classical*: They involve most of the points mentioned in the evaluation, but one or two symptom complexes are predominantly affected. One must strive to establish the main or predominant defect in fluency, comprehension, or repetition.
- *Danger of early evaluation of aphasias in strokes:* In an acute stroke, there is a core area of infarction/hemorrhage surrounded by edema and an area of ischemia. The latter two may gradually subside with therapy. Therefore, in strokes, the character of the aphasia may change; for example, in a nonfluent aphasia, initially comprehension may be affected. As the edema and ischemia subside, comprehension may improve, and the predominant defect of fluency becomes obvious. The optimal time of evaluation of an aphasia in strokes is between 2 and 4 weeks depending on the severity of the lesion.

There are many different names for aphasic syndromes, but most have commonly occurring neurologic signs; that is, they fit into a symptom complex **(Table 3.1)**.

TABLE 3.1: Analysis of aphasic syndromes.

					Reading		
	Sp Sp	Comp	Rpt	Nam	Aloud	Comp	Writing
Broca's	NF	+	–	+/–	–	+	–
Wernicke's	F	—	–	–	–	–	+
Conduction	F	+	—	–	–	+	+
Transcortical motor aphasia	NF	+	+	+	+	+	+/–
Transcortical sensory aphasia	F	–	+ echolalia	–	–	–	–
Anomic (nominal)	F	+	+	—	–	–	+

(Comp: comprehension; F: fluent; Nam: naming; NF: nonfluent; Rpt: repetition; Sp Sp: spontaneous speech; +: not affected; –: affected; —: main affected symptom complex)

Characteristics of Aphasias

The characteristics of the various aphasias will be enumerated based on the six points of bedside evaluation.

Broca's Aphasia (Table 3.1, First Row)

The lesion is usually an infarct in the left middle cerebral artery (MCA) territory involving the left inferior frontal gyrus and is anterior to the sylvian fissure **(Figs. 3.2A and B)**.

1. *Spontaneous speech*: Nonfluent, sparse output, best described as "telegraphic" or "SMS" speech. There is dysprosody with considerable effort in initiating speech which is dysarthric.
2. *Comprehension*: This is much better than spontaneous speech. The meaning is full with decreased phrase length—telegraphic or SMS speech.
3. *Repetition*: This is always abnormal and in proportion to the nonfluent spontaneous speech.
4. *Naming*: This is abnormal because of the nonfluency but relatively good compared to the lack of spontaneous speech. The patient may not be able to name the object but is able to mime its use/function.
5. *Reading*: Reading out aloud is very difficult but reading with comprehension is relatively better.
6. *Writing*: The handwriting is very poor but there are no spelling mistakes.

In Broca's aphasia, the involvement of the motor association areas for the face, lips, tongue, and oropharynx interferes with the formation of motor speech patterns explaining the main feature of nonfluency. Secondly, larger infarcts will involve the neighboring face and hand cortical motor areas.

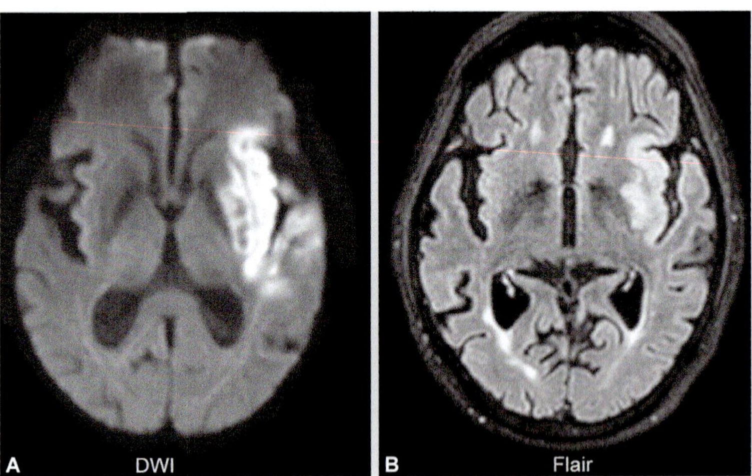

FIGS. 3.2A AND B: MRI of left MCA infarct producing Broca's aphasia. (A) DWI; (B) FLAIR.
(DWI: diffusion-weighted imaging; FLAIR: fluid attenuated inversion recovery; MCA: middle cerebral artery; MRI: magnetic resonance imaging)

Hence, a dense faciobrachial involvement in Broca's aphasia implies a poor prognosis for recovery.

Wernicke's Aphasia (Table 3.1, Second Row)

The lesion is usually posterior to the sylvian fissure. Hence, in the majority of cases, there is no hemiparesis. The lesion which is usually an infarct involves the left posterior temporal gyrus **(Fig. 3.3)**.

1. *Spontaneous speech*: The speech is fluent and may be augmented with various paraphasia producing a "logorrhea". The speech is melodic but meaningless with many literal or phonemic paraphasia and neologistics. In extreme cases, there is jargon aphasia.
2. *Comprehension*: This is abnormal and together with the fluent speech is one of the main features of Wernicke's aphasia (WA). This markedly reduces the ability of the patient to communicate. In some patients with WA, there is a striking lack of concern which may be replaced by paranoid behavior. As these patients usually do not have any hemiparesis, there is a danger of being initially evaluated by a psychiatrist for acute psychosis. The true worth of a psychiatrist is one who can detect the organicity of a patient with WA, as a grossly abnormal speech is rarely a presenting symptom of acute psychosis.
3. *Repetition*: This is impaired in proportion to spontaneous fluent speech and abnormal comprehension.
4. *Naming*: This is grossly abnormal. The patient may fail to name the object or gives a paraphasic response.

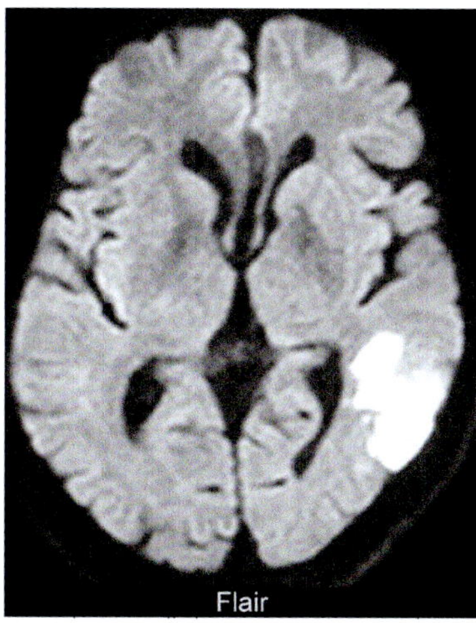

FIG. 3.3: MRI showing a left MCA infarct producing a Wernicke's aphasia.

Note: This infarct extends deep enough to produce a homonymous field of vision defect.

(FLAIR: fluid attenuated inversion recovery; MCA: middle cerebral artery; MRI: magnetic resonance imaging)

5. *Reading*: This is also abnormal and parallels the disturbance in spontaneous speech.
6. *Writing*: Handwriting is neat, but it lacks meaning and there are spelling mistakes.

A large infarct producing WA may extend deep into the subcortical area and involve the temporoparietal optic radiation. Hence, with a WA, it is a good practice to check for a homonymous hemianopia as the presence of one indicates a poor prognosis. As the patient's comprehension is affected, this is best achieved by a threat response in the contralateral temporal field of vision.

Conduction Aphasia (Table 3.1, Third Row)

The lesion in CAs involves Wernicke's loop connecting Wernicke's area to Broca's. The lesion is, therefore, subcortical involving the anteroinferior part of the parietal lobe with variable findings of hemiparesis or hemisensory defects. The true nature of this aphasia is usually seen during the recovery phase of a subcortical infarct.

1. *Spontaneous speech*: The speech is fluent but less than Wernicke's aphasia (WA) and more than Broca's aphasia (BA).
2. *Comprehension*: This is remarkably good and may be adequate for normal conversation.
3. *Repetition*: This is grossly abnormal and the main feature of this aphasia.
4. *Naming*: This is abnormal, but the patient may be able to mime the function as comprehension is remarkably preserved.
5. *Reading*: Reading aloud is abnormal but reading for comprehension may be relatively better. In some cases, reading for comprehension is affected indicating a posterior extension of the infarct to involve the angular gyrus.
6. *Writing*: Handwriting is untidy. In contrast to BA, spellings are poor with omissions, reversals, or substitution of letters.

Many patients with CA have buccofacial or limb apraxia, but body movements are spared.

A global or total aphasia involves the language circuit from Broca's area to Wernicke's area. It is usually due to a large infarct involving the entire left MCA territory or a large intracerebral hemorrhage. During recovery, features of a BA or WA may predominate, depending on the site of the lesion.

Transcortical Aphasias (Table 3.1, Fourth and Fifth Rows)

Transcortical aphasias are due to deep white matter lesions of the dominant hemisphere which spare the main language areas, i.e., Broca's and Wernicke's areas, as well as Wernicke's loop. These lesions separate the main language area from other cortical areas. If these lesions are in the association cortex of the frontal lobe, anterior or inferior to Broca's area, they result in a transcortical motor aphasia (TMA).

Transcortical motor aphasia: The characteristic features of TMA are similar to BA but with intact repetition.

Transcortical sensory aphasia (TSA): This is rare and results from subcortical white matter lesions in the temporo-occipital area. The most prominent feature of TSA is echolalia with other features similar to WA. There is a case report of a female patient who tried to commit suicide by putting her head in a gas oven. During her recovery phase, she had features of TSA. Her echolalia was so prominent that if the treating physician said, "roses are red", she would complete the rhyme by saying "roses are red, violets are blue, sugar is sweet and so are you". Thus, the main feature of transcortical aphasias, both motor and sensory, is intact repetition **(Flowchart 3.1)**.

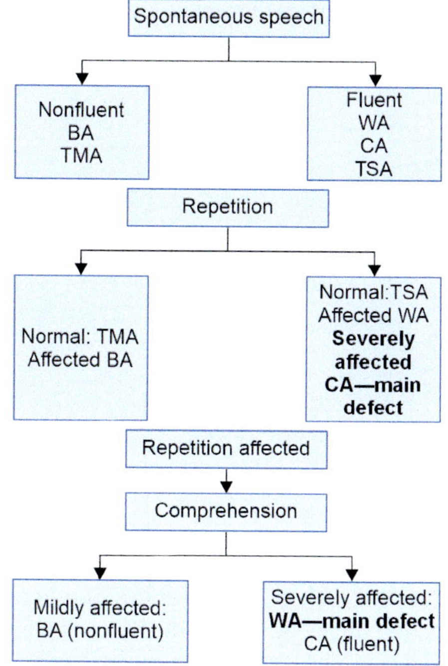

FLOWCHART 3.1: Analysis of aphasias.

(BA: Broca's aphasia; CA: conduction aphasia; TMA/TSA: transcortical motor/sensory aphasia; WA: Wernicke's aphasia)

Anomic Aphasia (Table 3.1, Sixth Row)

This is also known as nominal aphasia. The main defect is naming. As mentioned earlier, this type of aphasia lacks the localizing value of the other types of aphasic syndromes. The lesion usually is in the vicinity of the angular gyrus (area of concepts) but could be diffusely in the frontal, temporal, or parietal areas. It is seen in nonaphasic conditions like acute confusional states, dementias, or metabolic disorders. It is also frequently seen in the intensive care unit during recovery from coma.

Detecting Handedness in an Aphasic Patient

At times, a patient is admitted in a drowsy and unresponsive state or is aphasic. In such a situation, it is important to know the dominant hand. In India, this problem is further accentuated because we eat with our right hand and toilet hygiene is performed with the left hand. Thus, many left-handed individuals are forced to write with their right hands. In these situations, the dominant hand is identified by observing the nail bed of the thumb **(Figs. 3.4A and B)**. On the dominant side, the nail bed is broader and is a more of a "squarish U shape" compared to the nondominant side which has a more gentle U-shape. I do not know what the effect of typing on the mobile phone with both thumbs will have on this observation.

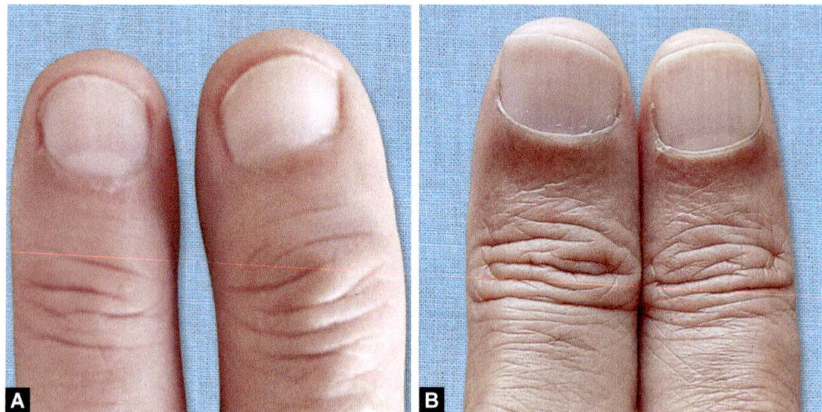

FIGS. 3.4A AND B: (A) The author's thumbs. Note that the right thumb nail bed is broader and more "squarish". (B) In a left-handed individual, a similar difference is also obvious.

I have my variation on this issue. Many Indians wear a ring on their left index and ring fingers. If so, try and remove the ring from the left side and put it on the respective finger on the right. If you have great difficulty in negotiating the ring across the proximal interphalangeal joint, then that is the dominant hand because the girth of the fingers is larger on the dominant side. This is true for individuals who use one hand predominantly in their day-to-day work or sporting activity. In individuals who work on computers and do touch typing, this difference may not be that obvious unless they play a sport like tennis or badminton regularly.

FRONTAL LOBE RELEASE REFLEXES

Automatic grasping and groping responses are normally present in neonates and disappear approximately after 1 year of age. In adults, these reflexes are inhibited by the frontal lobe. Hence, these responses reappear in adults when there is acquired brain damage, particularly to the frontal lobes. Therefore, these reflexes are known as frontal lobe release reflexes. They are commonly seen in patients with dementia, metabolic encephalopathy, traumatic brain injury (TBI), and hydrocephalus. Since diffuse cerebral dysfunction is associated with all these conditions, these reflexes have no localizing value. The most frequently tested frontal lobe release reflexes are the pout/snout, mouthing, and the palmomental response.

Pout/Snout reflex: A brisk pout-like protrusion of the lips occurs when the center of the upper lip is tapped. This resembles a pig's snout, hence the name.

Mouthing reflex: The patient opens his mouth when the corner of the mouth is stroked, as if he wants to bite an object.

Palmomental reflex: An involuntary contraction of the mentalis muscle of the chin occurs when the ipsilateral thenar eminence is stimulated. The peculiarity of this reflex is that the stimulus is far away from the site of response. A few salient facts about this reflex are as follows:
- It may be present in normal people, the prevalence varying widely. However, it is easily fatigable in normal people.
- Merely testing for the presence or absence of this reflex lacks sensitivity and specificity.
- There is no increase in prevalence with age.
- An abnormal palmomental reflex is less fatigable with nervous disease compared to normal people.
- It has no localizing value, even if unilateral, and merely alerts the examiner of some cerebral pathology.
- If a strong nonfatigable and easily repeatable contraction of the mentalis muscle is obtained by stimulation of areas other than the thenar eminence, the reflex is more likely to be significant for brain damage.
- It usually occurs in strokes, multiple sclerosis, motor neuron disease, TBI, tumors, Down's syndrome, acquired immunodeficiency syndrome (AIDS), and Parkinson's disease.

The other frontal lobe release reflexes of some clinical significance are as follows:
Tonic grasp reflex: On attempting to shake hands with the patient, the latter is unable to release his grasp; that is, the reaction outlasts the stimulus. This reflex is of localizing value only if it is unilateral and indicates a lesion of the thalamus or striatum.

Perseveration of grasping and groping: After shaking hands with the examiner, the patient again grasps for the examiner's hand or gropes for his clothes. This reflex is usually bilateral and occurs with diffuse cerebral cortical dysfunction.

Grasp reflex of the foot: This has the same evolution as the tonic grasp reflex of the hand and in adults is always pathological. On stroking the sole of the foot near the ball of the great toe, there is a flexion–adduction movement of all the toes enabling the patient to hold an object thrust between the toes for 15–30 seconds.

Tonic plantar reflex: On stroking the lateral part of the foot, the plantar flexion of the toes persists even after the stimulation has ended. It is one of the earliest signs of a frontal lobe lesion, more commonly with a frontal lobe tumor and less commonly with a hemorrhage. It is elicited even before the plantar response becomes extensor. The lesion is usually in or around the supplementary motor area (precentral gyrus).

RECOMMENDED ARTICLES

1. Benson DF, Geschwind N. Aphasias and Related Disorders: A clinical approach. In M-Marsel Mesulam (Ed). Principles of behavioural neurology. Contemporary neurology series, vol 26. FA Davis Company, Philadelphia; 1985. pp. 193-238.
2. Block JE. Thumb down on left-handedness. Letters to the editor. N Engl. J Med. 1974;291:307.
3. Haymaker W. Motor, sensory, reflex and related disturbances of cerebral cortical and subcortical origin. In Haymaker W (Ed). Bing's Local diagnosis in Neurological Diseases. St. Louis: The C. V. Mosby Company; 1969. pp. 329-48.

CHAPTER 4

Cranial Nerve 1: The Olfactory Nerve—the Neglected Cranial Nerve

I call the olfactory nerve the neglected cranial nerve because postgraduates, during their training years, and practicing neurologists hardly ever examine it. I do confess that in all my 50 years of practice, I am guilty of the same. There are many causes of bilateral anosmia **(Box 4.1)**.

Recently, studies have shown that olfactory loss is a good biomarker in Alzheimer's disease (AD) and Parkinson's disease (PD). It predicts the loss of gray matter in the hippocampus and therefore predicts which individual with minimal cognitive impairment-amnestic (MCI-a) will develop AD. An interesting point is that most of these individuals are unaware of this loss. Secondly, testing for olfactory loss becomes a cost-effective way to predict the future development of AD compared to amyloid positron emission tomography (PET) scan or cerebrospinal fluid (CSF) Aβ40/42 ratio–tests which are invasive, exorbitantly expensive, and, most importantly, not available to us. A progression of olfactory loss also predicts a progression of hippocampal neuronal loss. Thus, the loss of smell, which begins in MCI-a, progresses throughout the course of AD. In PD, loss of sense of smell either precedes or is well established by the time of diagnosis. It is less impaired in tremorgenic PD compared to the akinetic rigid variant. Thus, olfactory loss predicts cognitive dysfunction and is likely to be an important biomarker in many other neurodegenerative disorders.

Olfactory loss may also raise some management and safety issues in such patients. In addition to odor recognition, smell is necessary for appreciating the flavor of food. The aroma of coffee or the cooking of your favorite meal

BOX 4.1 | Causes of bilateral anosmia.

- Common cold
- Minor or major head trauma
- Exposure to pesticides, solvents, and cocaine
- *Medications*: Antibiotics, antidepressants, and certain cardiac drugs
- *Neurodegenerative conditions*: Parkinson's disease (PD) and Alzheimer's disease (AD)
- *Rare causes*: Epilepsy, type 2 diabetes, systemic lupus erythematosus (SLE), Sjögren's syndrome

stimulates your appetite. Loss of smell may lead to decrease in appetite and so called "unexplained" weight loss. At times, the patient may not be able to smell spoilt food and consuming it may lead to health issues. They may not be able to smell smoke or leaking gas, creating safety issues. Fortunately, in India, because of our strong family ties and respect for the elderly, such patients are practically never left alone and have a caregiver.

In recent times, loss of sense of smell was a prominent feature of coronavirus disease 2019 (COVID-19) infection and there are speculations about the direct spread of the virus to the brain through the olfactory apparatus.

Dysosmia is defined as an unpleasant or foul smell. This may be triggered or spontaneous. Tobacco, coffee, petrol, or strong attars/perfumes are common triggers. It occurs commonly following upper respiratory tract viral infection, chronic sinus disease, and cerebral trauma or is idiopathic. An important cause of dysosmia for the neurologist is the olfactory aura in mesial temporal lobe epilepsy. When I was the registrar in the neurology department of JJ Hospital, I distinctly remember a young patient who was standing on the balcony of his home, when he suddenly got dysosmia. He thought that the foul smell was due to a rotting plant and threw the pot out. Fortunately, no one got hurt. As he tried to go back, he got a generalized convulsion. Investigations revealed a glioma in the right temporal lobe. A point to remember is that in seizure disorders, the dysosmia lasts for a brief period whereas in other etiologies it can last for 5 minutes to hours.

Unilateral anosmia is uncommon and often overlooked as the cranial nerve is never examined. What is the clinical situation in which you should examine the olfaction in each nostril? This clinical situation is in a patient complaining of de novo headache associated with a unilateral progressive loss of vision. If there is ipsilateral anosmia, then one can safely make a diagnosis of olfactory groove meningioma and refer the patient for neuroimaging. With the advent of magnetic resonance imaging (MRI), one may argue that this has become a superfluous exercise. In my opinion, there is a certain amount of joy in making a clinical diagnosis and getting it confirmed by neuroimaging. Remember, the neuroradiologist has a fairly good idea as to which neurologist has a good clinical acumen with a high "hit" rate on MRI as against a mediocre one who does MRI as part of a defensive practice.

I hope with this account of olfaction, the olfactory nerve will find its rightful place in your clinical examination and is no longer the "neglected" cranial nerve.

RECOMMENDED ARTICLES

1. Devere R. Smell and taste in clinical neurology: 5 new things. Neurol Clin Pract. 2012;2:208-14.
2. Woo CC, Miranda B, Sathishkumar M, Dehkordi-Vakil F, Yassa MA, Leon M. Overnight olfactory enrichment using an odorant diffuser improves memory and modifies the uncinated fasciculus in older adults. Front Neurosci. 2023;17:1200448.

CHAPTER 5

Cranial Nerve 2: The Optic Nerve

The optic nerve is one of the most important cranial nerves as it serves one of our very precious senses—vision. There is a particular sequence of examination of the optic nerve: (1) Acuity of vision (A/V), (2) field of vision (F/V), (3) color vision, (4) the afferent pathway of the pupillary reflex, and (5) fundus examination.

ACUITY OF VISION TESTING

The A/V is accurately measured by Snellen's chart for the last 160 years. Nowadays, handheld Snellen's charts are available in various Indian languages and acuity can be measured when these are held at a specified distance.

FIELD OF VISION TESTING

This is tested by the confrontation method where the examiner's hands are held at an equidistant position from the patient. The patient closes one eye and has to answer whether the examiner's hand is waving or steady, held like a fist, or in a V for victory sign. This requires patience, both from the examiner and from the patient, as it is cumbersome and time consuming.

I have a rather simple confrontation method for screening the F/V. Stand in front of the eye of the patient that you want to examine with your hands held as shown in **Figure 5.1**.

Note that the hand reflecting the nasal F/V of the patient should be closer to your face than the one reflecting the temporal F/V. Then ask the patient, "do you see my face clearly or my hands (usually the one reflecting the temporal F/V)?" If the patient has a central scotoma, he/she will respond by stating that your face is not clear **(Fig. 5.2)**.

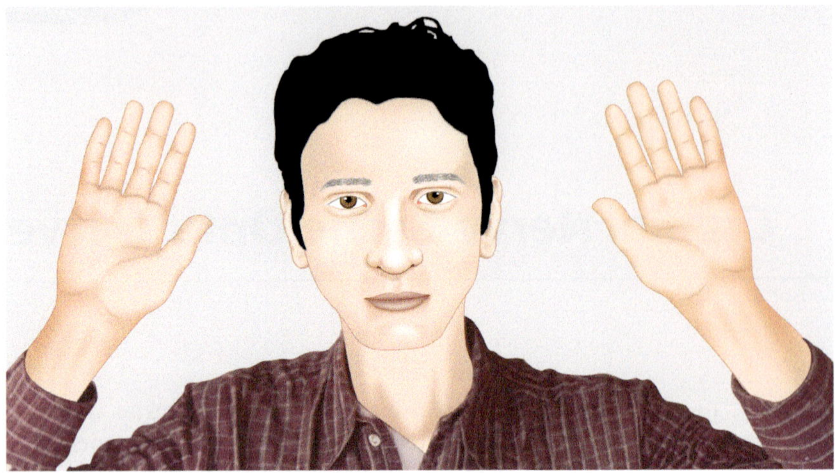

FIG. 5.1: Position adopted for testing field of vision (F/V).

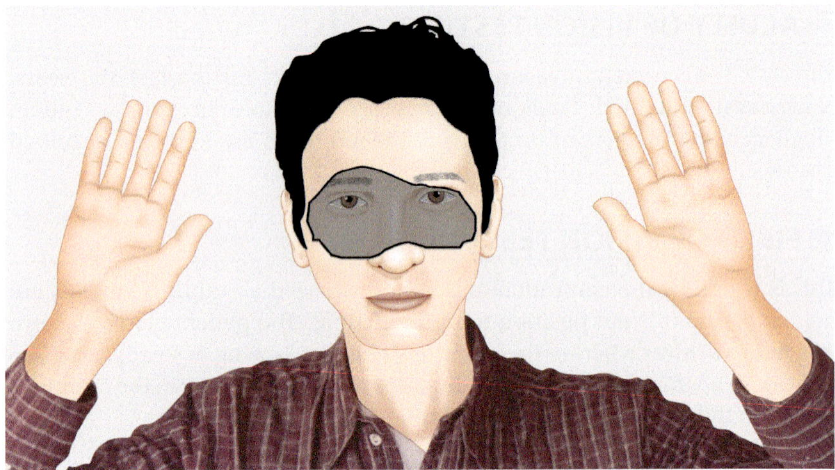

FIG. 5.2: Patient's response for a central or centrocecal scotoma.

On the other hand, if there is a homonymous hemianopia, the patient will complain of blurring or inability to see your hand in the temporal F/V with a clear-cut vertical line of demarcation **(Fig. 5.3)**.

Lastly, if the patient has an altitudinal F/V defect, he/she will complain of inability to see either the upper or lower part of your face and hands **(Fig. 5.4)**.

This is a simple screening method and gives quick results. Of course, you will have to establish the type of F/V defect by doing a formal F/V charting. Nevertheless, this method has held me in good stead at the bedside.

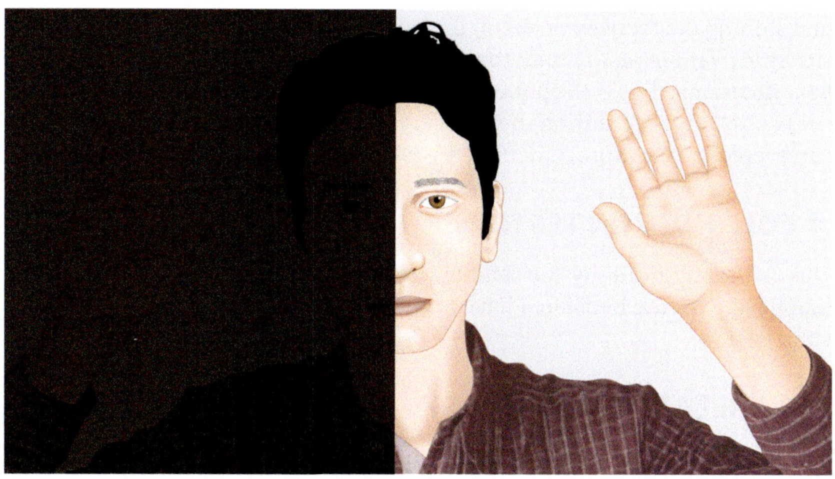

FIG. 5.3: Patient's response for a left homonymous hemianopia.

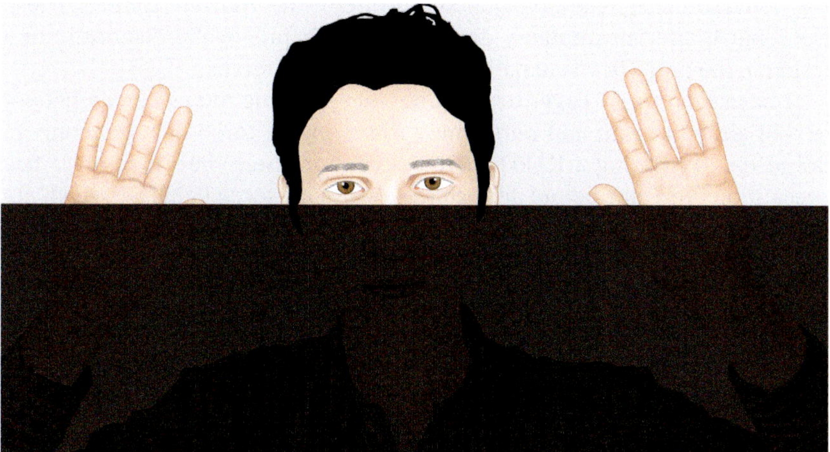

FIG. 5.4: Patient's response for an altitudinal field of vision (F/V) defect.

Another useful tip for testing the F/V is in the cases of hemianopia. I was examining a patient with a left posterior cerebral artery infarct and was about to do a fundus examination. As was my habit, I was in the temporal field of the patient and directed the beam of the ophthalmoscope toward the pupil to visualize the disc. As soon as I did this, the patient said that he could see the light now. This observation of the patient gave me the idea of using the macular beam of the ophthalmoscope to examine the temporal F/V in cases of homonymous hemianopia. This can be done by holding your ophthalmoscope about 6 inches away from the lateral canthus of the eye and shining the focused beam on the pupil. Then move the ophthalmoscope slowly forward in an arc until the patient says that he can see the light. Make your notations; that is, the patient can see the beam at 90° (right in front of the eye) or at 75° or 45° during the recovery phase. This way, at the bedside you can even plot the improvement in the F/V on follow-up.

COLOR VISION TESTING

This is usually done by the Ishihara charts, which are now available as a mobile app. At the bedside, I have nothing to contribute regarding testing of color vision.

PUPILLARY LIGHT REFLEX

Since we Indians have dark irises, it is not easy to appreciate anisocoria from afar and even more difficult to appreciate the consensual light reflex by the conventional method described in books of clinical methods. In India, the swinging torch light test is an easy and cost-effective way of eliciting the consensual light reflex. One should be aware that an abnormal test, the relative afferent pupillary defect (RAPD), is practically diagnostic of a lesion in the anterior visual pathway, i.e., the optic nerve.

I have seen many eager resident doctors standing too close to a patient in a brightly lit room and performing the swinging torch light test, only to fail in demonstrating a RAPD. Hence, I caution them that there are a few precautions you take before performing a swinging torch light test, which are as follows:

- Darken the room considerably, so that the pupils dilate as much as possible, particularly in the elderly in whom the pupils are likely to be constricted. This simple maneuver may make the anisocoria more obvious.
- Do not stand too close to the patient as this inadvertently produces convergence and constricts the pupil further. Stand at least 14 inches away and slightly to the side of the suspected abnormal eye. Ask the patient to look at a blank surface, which is at least 5–6 feet away. Also, note that your torch light has a powerful beam.
- The latency between the direct and consensual light reflex is 200–500 m/sec. Hence, swing the torch light in a U-shaped fashion every 1–2 seconds **(Fig. 5.5)**. Directing the torch light beam into one eye for a longer period may produce a pupillary hippus and vitiates the test. Begin by shining the beam in the normal eye so that the RAPD is obvious when you swing the torch light into the abnormal eye.

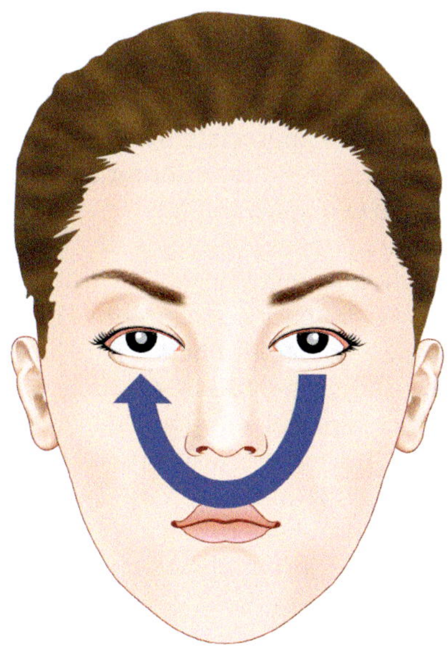

FIG. 5.5: Swinging torch light test: Move the torch in a U-shape manner starting with the normal eye.

FUNDUS EXAMINATION

Unlike an ophthalmologist, the neurologist does not have the luxury of dilated pupils to examine the fundus. The examination of the fundus with undilated pupils can only be achieved by constant practice, which should begin in your residency days. I remember my residency days when I struggled to see the optic disc, let alone the rest of the retina and blood vessels. During fundus examination, one should concentrate on the disc, the blood vessels, the macula, and the periphery of the retina. Standard textbooks have adequately described the changes seen in the blood vessels and retina in hypertension and diabetes. Here, I would like to give you a few tips during the fundus examination. Again, I would like to stress that you should do the fundus examination in a darkened room so as to dilate the pupils as much as possible. To keep the patient's gaze fixed, keep a zero-watt red or dark-blue bulb on a wall 3–4 ft away, and ask the patient to look at it in a darkened room. For the right eye of the patient, use your right eye and vice versa for the left.

Since the neurologist will be very close to the patient's face, a few courtesies must be observed for the patient's benefit and cooperation. My mentor, Professor NH Wadia, advised me very early in my career that if you have an

OPD in the afternoon, do not eat onions at lunch. Patients do not appreciate a doctor's mouth smelling of onions. Secondly, he told me, "before you begin your consultations, please wash your face and apply an eau de cologne/ after shave lotion". Patients do appreciate the aroma of a cologne. I did that and one of my patients, who was a reporter for Stardust, did comment that Dr Katrak was very fond of Old Spice cologne.

During fundus examination, one should study the disc for optic atrophy or early papilledema. When you have a pale disc, the question always arises whether it is primary or secondary optic atrophy. The answer is very easily obtained by observing the crisscross fibers of the lamina cribrosa. If these fibers are prominently seen in the middle of a pale disc, it is primary optic atrophy. But if these fibers are not sharply delineated and are blurred, it is secondary optic atrophy. The latter is also true for early papilledema except that the disc is not pale and the margins of the disc are not sharply defined. Another aspect is to look at the arteries as they cross the edge of the disc. When the disc is swollen as in papilledema, the arteries "disappear into a cloud" as they cross the edge of the swollen disc, only to reappear again. Gross papilledema is very easy to diagnose.

Secondly, during fundus examination, look closely for venous pulsations. If they are present, the intracranial pressure (ICP) is normal. If the ICP is elevated, the veins become turgid and nonpulsatile. A word of caution when you are looking for venous pulsations: They may not be appreciated in both eyes. While checking for venous pulsations, ask the patient to breathe normally. Out of respect for the doctor, many patients hold their breath when you are in close proximity, like the fundus examination. This raises the intrathoracic pressure, thereby abolishing venous pulsations. When looking for venous pulsations, I have made it a practice to ask the patient to breathe normally, once I have focused on a vein.

These are a few tips I can give resident doctors and young neurologists in order to extract the maximum information from a fundus examination. Achieving all this is not going to be easy, but practice makes perfect.

Once you have mastered these aspects of fundus examination, you can try and visualize the periphery of the retina with undilated pupils. This should only be attempted when you suspect a pathology like retinitis pigmentosa (RP) or perivenous sheathing (PVS) which are predominantly seen in the periphery of the retina. This is by no means easy but with a lot of practice it is achievable. Once you fix the beam on the optic disc, you hold the beam steady and ask the patient to look slightly medially—for the nasal part of the retina and slightly laterally for the temporal part. Similarly, you can see the upper and lower parts of the retina by asking the patient to look up and down, respectively. In this way, I have picked up cases of Refsum's disease with RP and Eales disease with PVS in our busy OPD at the JJ Hospital. Of course, in both these cases, a proper documentation was done by an ophthalmologist with dilated pupils. There is a great deal of joy when your clinical diagnosis with undilated pupils is confirmed by them with dilated pupils.

Lastly, any good ophthalmoscope has a macular beam: The smallest diameter beam. The easiest way to visualize the macula is to focus the macular beam on the optic disc and then ask the patient to look at the beam. This will focus the beam on the macula. If you follow these clinical tips, examination of the optic nerve will be very easy and fruitful.

CLINICAL APPROACH TO UNEXPLAINED VISUAL LOSS

When a patient complains of unexplained visual loss (UVL), the problem may be twofold: Either the patient has subnormal A/V with a normal examination or normal acuity but still complains of visual loss.

Step 1

The first step is to separate optical problems from neuroretinal problems. In order to do this, do a pinhole test. If the A/V improves, it is an optical problem. Refer the patient to an ophthalmologist for further evaluation. A classic example is refractory error. If the acuity does not improve, it is a neuroretinal problem.

Step 2

For a neuroretinal problem, do a swinging torch light test. This will detect either a presence or an absence of RAPD.

The common cause of RAPD is a unilateral optic nerve disease. Uncommonly, RAPD may be present in extensive retinal disease or in asymmetrical chiasmal compression.

Step 3

Patient has RAPD. Do a bedside F/V testing. This may either show (1) A nerve-fiber bundle type of defect or (2) a hemianopic defect.

Step 3A

Patient has RAPD. F/V testing shows nerve fiber bundle defect (NFBD) **(Fig. 5.6)**.

The various types of NFBD are: (1) Central or centrocecal scotoma, (2) altitudinal defect, (3) a concentric restriction of the F/V, and (4) an arcuate scotoma.

Also see **Figures 5.2 and 5.4**.

Central or centrocecal scotoma: It is a variety of nerve fiber bundle type of defect suggestive of optic neuritis **(Fig. 5.6A)**. It usually affects young women more than men and is a risk factor for the development of multiple sclerosis (MS) or other demyelinating disorders. In adults, it is usually unilateral but is commonly bilateral in children. The scotoma is due to the selective involvement of the maculopapillary bundle, which is lodged in the central part of the optic nerve. This is usually due to an inflammatory or a demyelinating

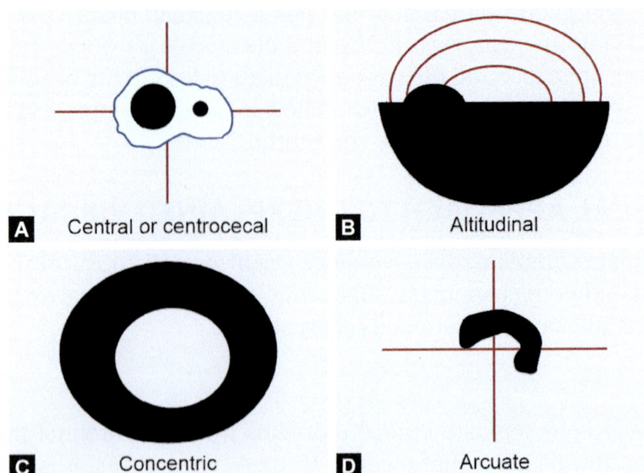

FIGS. 5.6A TO D: Various types of nerve fiber bundle defects. (A) Central or centrocecal; (B) Altitudinal; (C) Concentric; (D) Arcuate.

lesion and denotes a noncompressive pathology. It can progress rapidly over 2–5 days to total loss of vision. A peculiar feature of this optic neuritis is that orbital or retro-orbital pain can precede visual loss by 24–48 hours and that this pain is aggravated by eye movements. The term retrobulbar neuritis is reserved for posteriorly placed lesions of the optic nerve (behind the eyeball), and initially there is no optic disc pallor. An anteriorly placed lesion involving the optic disc produces swelling and exudates and is called papillitis. This is often confused with early papilledema. This problem is easily resolved by noting the A/V. If the drop in A/V is out of proportion to the swelling of the disc, it is papillitis, whereas with early papilledema, there is hardly any drop in the A/V.

Another uncommon variety of NFBD is an altitudinal defect **(Fig. 5.6B)**. The most common cause of this is glaucoma. In neurology, it is produced by an arteritic or nonarteritic branch occlusion of the retinal artery. However, it is the second most common NFBD in neuromyelitis optica (NMO). In a patient with an altitudinal F/V defect, papilledema is stated to be an essential finding in the early stages of ischemic optic neuropathy, and it is invariably a painless condition. These features help to differentiate it from a demyelinating disorder.

Concentric constriction of the F/V is also uncommon and is usually seen in postpapilledematous secondary optic atrophy **(Fig. 5.6C)**.

An arcuate scotoma is a variety of NFBD, occurring rarely in demyelinating disorders. It is due to the involvement of the arching arcuate fibers surrounding the maculopapillary bundle. If it is due to an ischemic lesion, it is a focal type of altitudinal defect **(Fig. 5.6D)**.

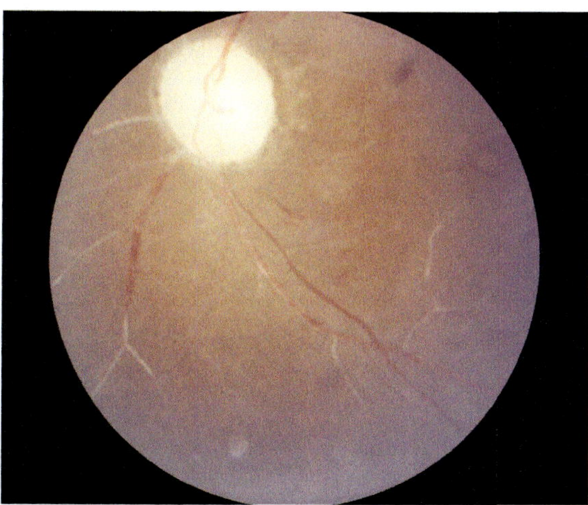

FIG. 5.7: Fundal photograph: Central retinal artery occlusion in a human immunodeficiency virus (HIV) positive individual. Note the pale disc and empty blood vessels.
Courtesy: Dr Phiroze Patel.

Optic nerve disease etiologies are as follows:
Demyelinating disorders: MS, NMO spectrum disorders (NMOSD), myelin oligodendrocyte glycoprotein antibody-associated disease (MOGAD).

Vascular disorders: Central retinal artery occlusion **(Fig. 5.7)**, anterior ischemic optic neuropathy, and amaurosis fugax.

Phacomatosis: Neurofibromatosis, tuberous sclerosis, and angiomatosis of retina and central nervous system—Von Hippel-Landau syndrome **(Figs. 5.8A and B)**.

Infections and infestations: Central nervous system tuberculosis (CNS TB), cytomegalovirus infection, and rarely neurocysticercosis **(Fig. 5.9)**.

Step 3B

Patient has RAPD. F/V testing shows a hemianopic defect.

The most common etiologies will be lesions of the junction of the optic nerve and chiasma producing a junctional scotoma.

Junctional scotoma: As I mentioned earlier, the majority of scotomas are due to noncompressive etiologies. An exception to the rule is the junctional scotoma **(Fig. 5.10)**. In this entity, the lesion is at the junction of the optic nerve with the chiasma producing an ipsilateral scotoma (as the name suggests) together with a contralateral quadrantic or hemianopic defect. The latter is because of the peculiar anatomy of the crossing nasal fibers, which form a loop at the lateral end of the chiasma and dip into the optic nerve.

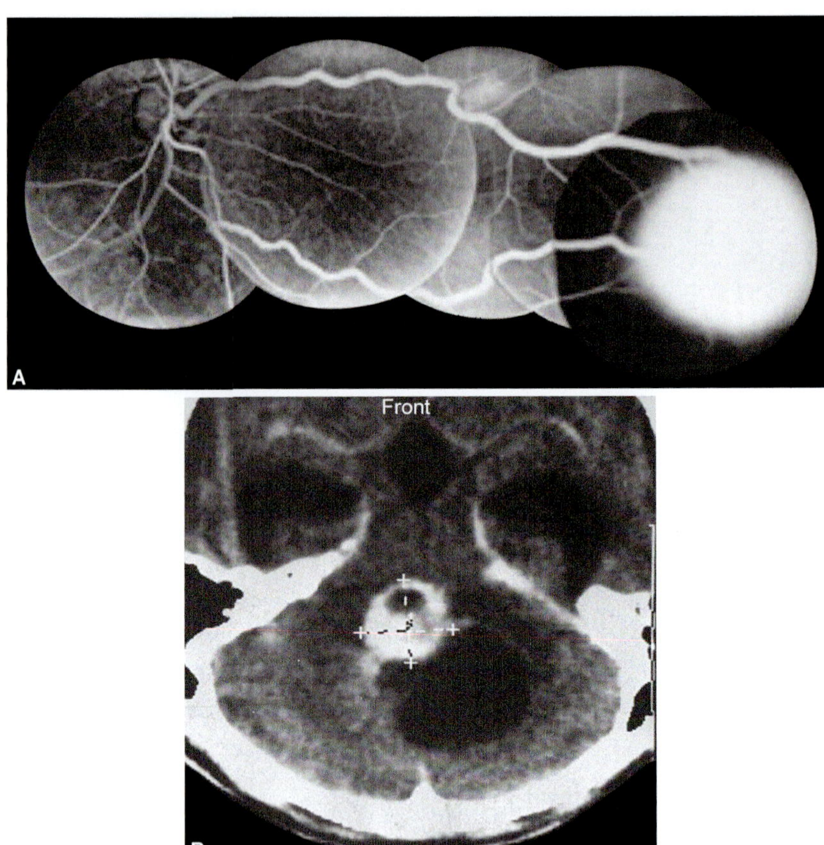

FIGS. 5.8A AND B: (A) Montage formed by a series of fundal photographs showing a peripheral angioma, in a patient with Von Hippel–Lindau syndrome; (B) Postcontrast computed tomography (CT) scan of the same patient showing a cerebellar hemangioblastoma.

Hence, in a patient with progressive unilateral visual loss, in whom an ipsilateral anosmia has been ruled out (see Chapter 4, olfactory nerve), please look closely for a contralateral temporal quadrantic or hemianopic defect. If present, a compressive etiology should be ruled out by neuroimaging. If the peculiar features of a junctional scotoma are not picked up early in the course of the problem, the patient is in danger of permanently losing vision in one eye.

Case Vignette

GP was a 34-year-old male patient who complained of progressive loss of vision in the right eye. He was diagnosed as a case of "retrobulbar neuritis" by an ophthalmologist and given several intraocular steroid injections. When he presented to me, he was totally blind in the right eye and had a left temporal

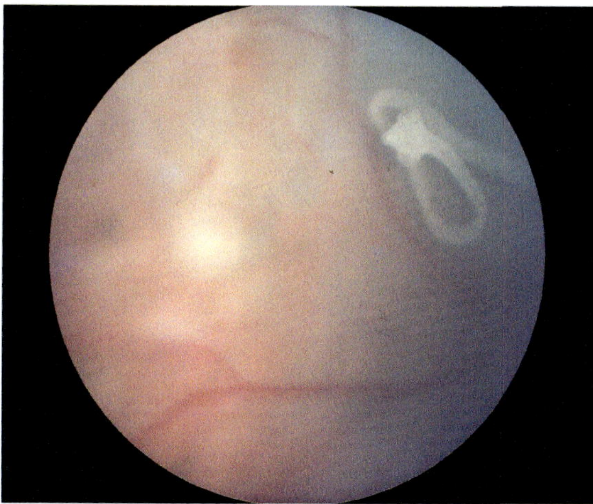

FIG. 5.9: Fundal photograph showing larvae of cysticercus in a patient with unilateral blindness and epilepsy.

Courtesy: Late Dr Kanti Modi.

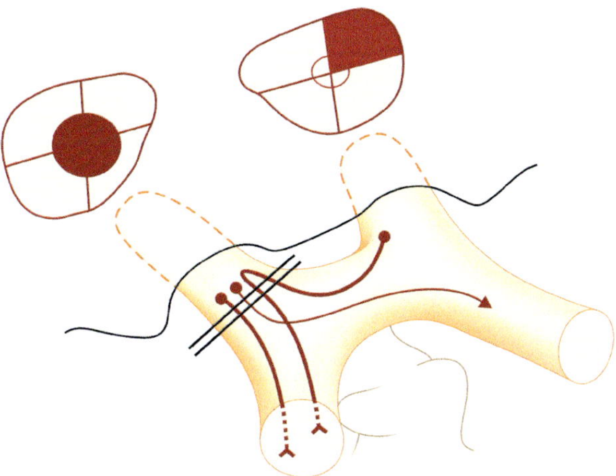

FIG. 5.10: Junctional scotoma. The site of the lesion is denoted by dual lines.

F/V defect. A computed tomography (CT) scan done in July 1988 showed a suprasellar pituitary macroadenoma producing a junctional scotoma **(Fig. 5.11)**. Unfortunately, the patient did not recover the vision in his right eye.

Lesions of the optic chiasma and tract can uncommonly produce a RAPD in combination with bitemporal hemianopic F/V defects which localize the lesion to the optic chiasma.

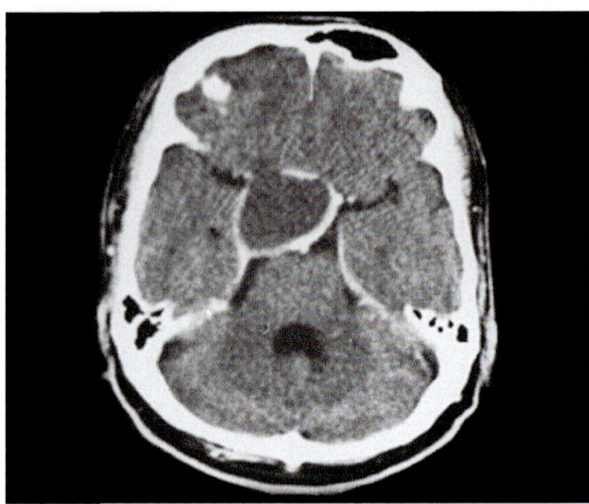

FIG. 5.11: Patient with right junctional scotoma due to pituitary macroadenoma.

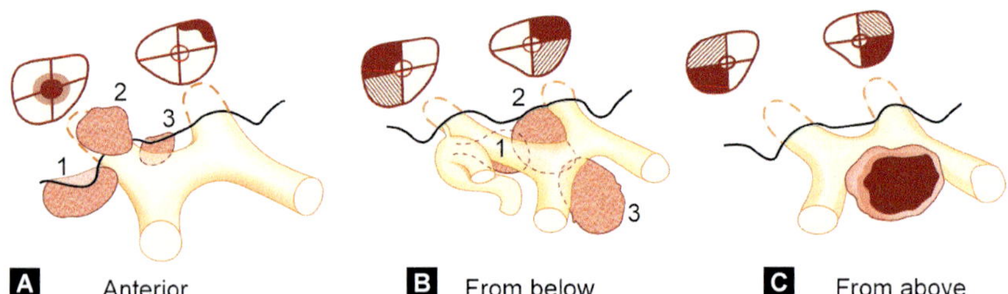

FIGS. 5.12A TO C: Various compressive lesions of the optic chiasma. Details are given in the text.

Lesions of the optic chiasma are usually due to compression from tumors. The compression may be either anteriorly, from below, or above **(Figs. 5.12A to C)**. Anterior compressive lesions are usually due to (1) sphenoidal ridge, (2) olfactory groove, or (3) tuberculum sella meningiomas. Compressions from below are usually due to (1) an aneurysm of the internal carotid artery, (2) pituitary adenoma, or (3) chordoma. Compressions from above are usually due to a craniopharyngioma.

The types of hemianopic defects produced by these tumors vary because of the crossing nasal fibers in the chiasma. The lower nasal fibers cross low and anteriorly and are involved early in compression from below. Thus, an early F/V defect due to a sellar mass is an upper temporal quadrantanopia. Similarly, the upper nasal fibers cross high and posteriorly and are compressed early by a suprasellar mass. Thus, a craniopharyngioma initially produces a lower temporal quadrantanopia.

Step 4

On the swinging torch light test, there is no RAPD. Rule out amblyopia (lazy eye due to abnormal visual development) and/or macular disease.

Etiologies of macular diseases are Tay-Sachs disease or sialidosis.

Step 5

If amblyopia and/or macular disease is ruled out, do F/V charting.
Various types of F/V defects that may be seen are as follows:

- *Tunnel vision*: Etiology-hysteria or malingering
- *Bilateral nerve fiber bundle type of defect*: Because the lesion is bilateral, there is no RAPD. Etiology-bilateral optic neuritis, usually in children in contrast to unilateral optic neuritis in adults
- *Bitemporal hemianopia*: Rare cases of central chiasmatic compression
- *Homonymous hemianopia*: This indicates a postchiasmal lesion of the optic radiation, from the optic peduncle to the occipital cortex **(Fig. 5.13)**. One must note that the hemianopic defect will vary depending on the site of involvement of the optic radiation as shown in **Figure 5.13**.

A homonymous hemianopia usually indicates a parenchymatous hemispheric lesion. I have only seen one case of a homonymous hemianopia due to compression from a convexity meningioma. Lastly, I would like to remind you that in cases of Wernicke's aphasia due to a large infarct, the

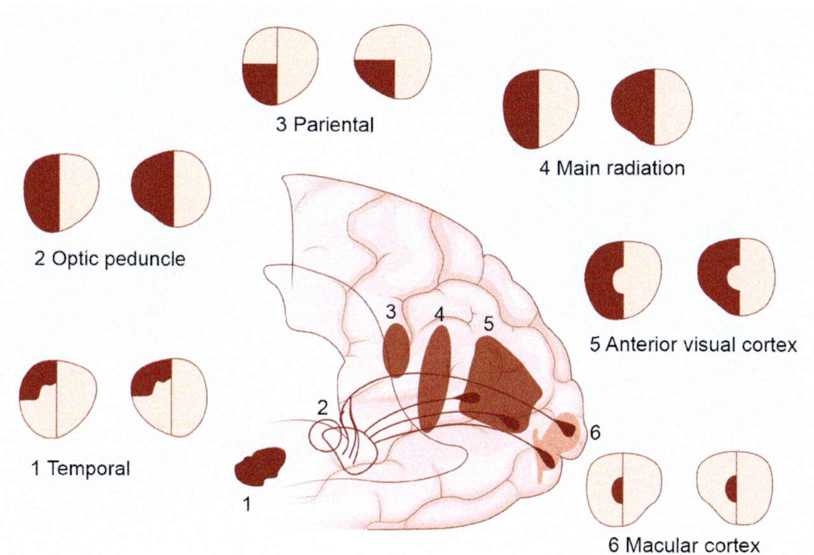

FIG. 5.13: Various types of homonymous hemianopic defects along the course of the optic radiation.

parietal optic radiation may be involved in the subcortical area and implies a poor prognosis for recovery.

RECOMMENDED ARTICLES

1. Prasad S, Galetta SL. Approach to a patient with acute visual loss. Neurol Clin Pract. 2012;2:14-23.
2. Nakajima H, Hosokawa T, Sugino M, Kimura F, Sugasawa J, Hanafusa T, et al. Visual field defects of optic neuritis in neuromyelitis optica compared with multiple sclerosis. BMC Neurol. 2010;10:45-50.

CHAPTER 6

Cranial Nerves 3, 4, and 6: The Oculomotor Cranial Nerves

Traditionally, the oculomotor (OCM), trochlear (TRL) and abducens (ABD) cranial nerves are examined together as the oculomotor cranial nerves. There are 12 muscles which move the eyeball and are divided into two groups: Eight recti and four oblique muscles.

The OCM cranial nerve innervates the medial rectus (MR), the superior rectus (SR), the inferior rectus (IR), and the inferior oblique (IO). Additionally, it innervates the levator palpebrae superioris and contributes to the parasympathetic innervation of the pupils. The TRL cranial nerve supplies only the superior oblique (SO) muscle and the ABD cranial nerve the lateral rectus (LR). Examination of the oculomotor nerves (OCMNs) involves examination of the external ocular movements (EOM), the pupillary constriction to light, and presence or absence of ptosis. Defects of the EOM involve ptosis, diplopia, and nystagmus.

A detailed description of localizing the paretic muscle in a case of diplopia is beyond the scope of this book, but certain anatomical facts are important in order to understand normal and abnormal EOM.

- The origin and attachments of the external ocular muscles are along the long axis of the orbit, which is approximately at 60° to each other in the skull, but the eyeballs in the primary position are frontally projected.
- Hence, only the MR/LR have their primary action of adduction and abduction, respectively, along the long axis of the muscles.
- The movement of the other muscles is complex. The SR and IR have their primary action of elevation and depression, respectively, only in abduction **(Fig. 6.1A)**. With the eyeball in the primary position, the SR will intort and the IR will extort the eyeball.
- The primary action (i.e., along the long axis of the muscle) of the SO is depression and of IO is elevation. This primary action can occur only with the adduction of the eyeball **(Fig. 6.1B)**. With the eyeball in the primary position, the SO intorts and the IO extorts the eyeball.
- **Figure 6.2 and Table 6.1** show the primary and secondary actions of the external ocular muscles.

It is easy to remember the primary action of the MR and LR. The action of the other muscles is complex. The primary action of the recti is in abduction, whereas the primary action of the obliques is in adduction **(Fig. 6.2)**. The easiest way to remember the primary action of the muscles,

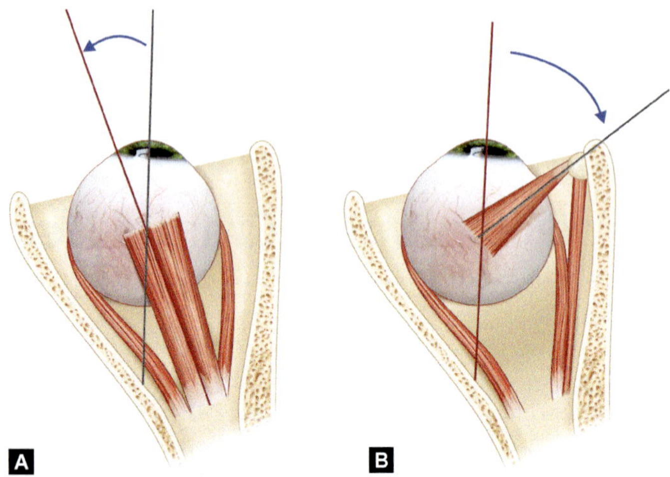

FIGS. 6.1A AND B: Dorsal view of the left eye. (A) Primary action of SR in abduction; (B) Primary action of SO in adduction.
(SO: superior oblique; SR: superior rectus)

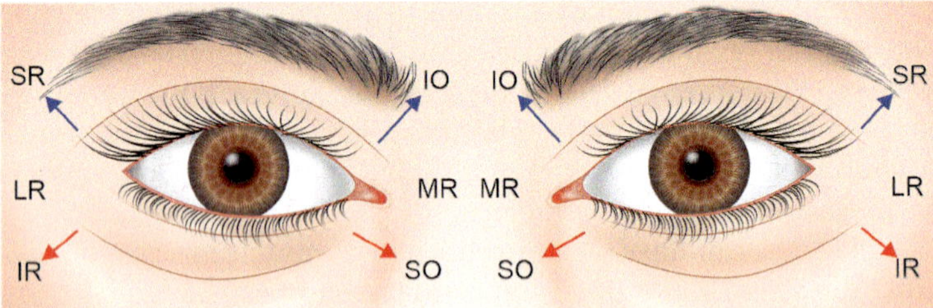

FIG. 6.2: Six points of references for the movements of the external ocular muscles.
(IO: inferior oblique; IR: inferior rectus; LR: lateral rectus; MR: medial rectus; SO: superior oblique; SR: superior rectus)

TABLE 6.1: Primary and secondary actions of the external ocular muscles.

	Primary action (along long axis)	Secondary action (primary position of eyeball)
MR	Adduction	–
LR	Abduction	–
SR	Elevation (in abduction)	Intorsion
IR	Depression (in abduction)	Extortion
SO	Depression (in adduction)	Intorsion
IO	Elevation (in adduction)	Extortion

(IO: inferior oblique; IR: inferior rectus; LR: lateral rectus; MR: medial rectus; SO: superior oblique; SR: superior rectus) which move the eyeball in the vertical plane, is as follows: If you ask the patient to look toward his/her nOSe, you are testing the Obliquus Superior. The primary action of the rest of EOM then falls into place.

ERRORS DURING CLINICAL EXAMINATION OF EXTERNAL OCULAR MOVEMENTS

At times, an overenthusiastic resident doctor goes too close to the patient to examine the EOM. This produces convergence of the eyes and during examination at the extremes of lateral movements elicits "false" nystagmus. When examining EOM, always keep your finger at least 14 inches away to maintain a conjugate position of the eyes.

One must always maintain binocular vision of the patient when testing EOM. Do not go beyond the range of horizontal adduction/abduction. If you do so, then the adducting eye is "blinded" and again you get nystagmus in the abducting eye. The "blinding" of the adducting eye is easily possible if the patient has deep-set eyes or high bridge of the nose **(Fig. 6.3A)**. The best

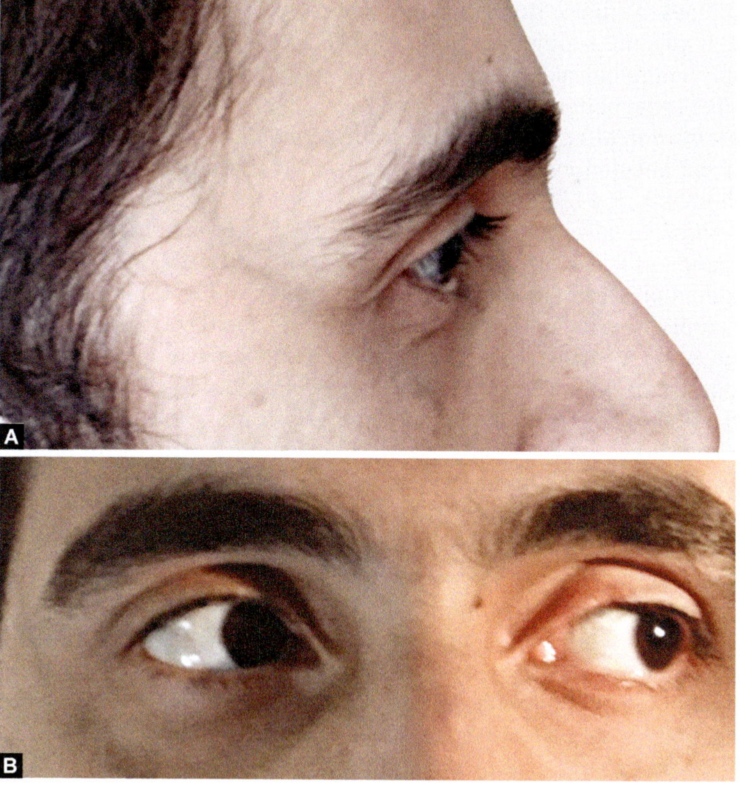

FIGS. 6.3A AND B: (A) The patient has a high bridge of the nose. (B) Note no reflection of the torchlight in the "blinded" adducting eye.

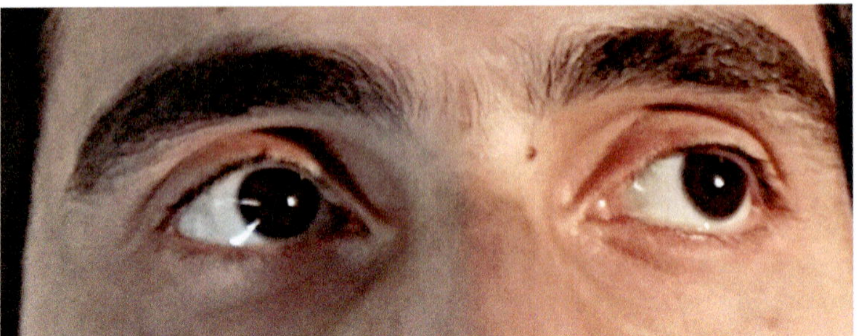

FIG. 6.4: The reflection of the torchlight in both eyes denotes binocular vision.
Note: This is the same patient as in Figure 6.3. The degree of adduction is less in his right eye.

way to confirm binocular vision is to ask the patient to follow a torch light and look for the reflection of it in the pupils **(Figs. 6.3B and 6.4)**.

Tips to be followed during the history elicitation and examination in a case presenting with diplopia are:

- Remember that diplopia is always sudden.
- Q: Does the diplopia disappear on covering either eye?
  A: If yes, the problem is neurological. If no, then the problem is local ophthalmological.
- What is the pattern of separation?
  Horizontal: MR or LR involved. If the separation increases on adduction of the affected eye, the MR is involved. If the separation increases on abduction, the LR is involved.
  Vertical: Involvement of SR, IR, SO, or IO. If the separation increases on abduction in the affected eye, the recti are involved and if it increases in adduction, the oblique muscles are involved (see **Fig. 6.1**). Put differently, if vertical separation increases on looking to the side of the paretic muscle, the recti are involved and if it increases on looking away from the paretic muscle, the oblique muscles are involved. In addition, if there is a head tilt to one side, the contralateral SO is the paretic muscle. Kindly note that in SO palsy, the head tilt must be corrected before examining for diplopia as the head tilt is a compensatory mechanism to avoid diplopia.
- Q: Is the diplopia worse on distant or near vision?
  A: Diplopia on horizontal + distant vision is suggestive of an LR palsy
  Diplopia on horizontal + near vision: Failure of convergence in neurodegeneration (common) or an isolated MR palsy (a rarity).
- Fluctuations or change in character of diplopia, either horizontal or vertical, is suggestive of myasthenia gravis (MG).
- Fluctuating diplopia with change in voice, difficulty in coughing, swallowing, or breathing is again suggestive of MG.
- Diplopia with pain on ocular movements is suggestive of microvascular disease—diabetes or giant cell arteritis. The latter may have headaches and jaw claudication during mastication.

- Torsional movements of the eyeball are difficult to pick up. However, watching the movement of a horizontally placed conjunctival vessel will make torsional movements easier to see. This becomes important when you want to judge the integrity of the trochlear nerve in the presence of a OCM nerve palsy. Since adduction (MR) is not possible, the primary action of the SO, i.e., depression, is not possible. But when the patient is instructed to look toward the nose, a small intorsion of the eye indicates the integrity of the SO and hence the trochlear nerve.

INVOLVEMENT OF THE OCULOMOTOR NERVES: A SIMPLIFIED APPROACH

Involvement of the Oculomotor (OCM) Cranial Nerve

There are six sites at which the oculomotor nerve can be involved. The important point to remember is the additional associated deficits, which are unique to each site.

1. *Nuclear lesion in the midbrain results in a unilateral OCM nerve palsy with a contralateral SR palsy*: This is because the SR muscle is innervated by the contralateral medial subnucleus of the OCM nerve. In addition, there may be bilateral ptosis because of the involvement of the caudally placed midline subnucleus supplying the levator palpebrae superioris bilaterally. Pure nuclear lesions in the midbrain are rare and usually accompanied by other midbrain signs.
2. *A fascicular lesion within the midbrain can occur at two sites-dorsal and ventral midbrain*: In the dorsal midbrain, there is a unilateral OCM nerve palsy with a contralateral rubrodentate tremor because of the involvement of the red nucleus—Benedikt syndrome. In the ventral midbrain, there is a unilateral OCM nerve palsy with a contralateral hemiplegia as the lesion involves the fascicular part of the OCM nerve near the crux cerebri—Weber syndrome.
3. *Lesions in the subarachnoid space*: In a OCM nerve palsy with pupillary involvement, it is prudent to rule out a compression from a posterior communicating (PCom) artery aneurysm. In diabetic OCM nerve palsy, only 50% have pupillary involvement (see later in the discussion of anisocoria). However, a majority of patients will have pain on movement of the paretic muscles (neurogenic claudication of the paretic muscle). In tubercular meningitis (TBM), the OCM nerve may be involved together with the optic nerve in basal exudates.
4. In cavernous sinus involvement, the OCM, TRL, and ABD nerves are involved together with the first division of the trigeminal nerve. As the oculosympathetic fibers travel to the eye together with the first division of the trigeminal nerve, they are involved producing congestion of the eye.
5. *Superior orbital fissure*: This structure is practically anterior to the cavernous sinus, and therefore the features are similar to those of cavernous sinus involvement.

6. *Within the orbit*: Again, the findings are similar to cavernous sinus involvement but in addition the optic nerve may be involved. If the etiology is a mass lesion, there will be an exophthalmos.

Involvement of the Trochlear (TRL) Cranial Nerve

Isolated TRL cranial nerve palsy is relatively rare. In children, it is usually congenital. A word of caution: The head tilt in children with congenital TRL nerve palsy may be misdiagnosed as torticollis.

In adults, it is usually trauma. The TRL cranial nerve is the only cranial nerve that emerges from the dorsal aspect of the brainstem at the level of the superior colliculus. As a consequence, it has a long intracranial course and is therefore prone to trivial trauma.

Involvement of the Abducens (ABD) Cranial Nerve

In children, the abducens nerve may be involved in two syndromes. The Möbius syndrome involves bilateral ABD and facial nerve palsies. The Duane syndrome is usually unilateral. It is detected when the gaze is in the direction of the paralyzed LR. Note that the patient does not complain of diplopia as the lesion is congenital. A key sign of this syndrome is retraction of the globe and narrowing of the palpebral fissure on adduction of the eye on the abnormal side which returns to normal in the primary position.

The abducens nucleus may be involved in vascular lesions of the pons:

Foville syndrome: ABD and facial nerve palsy with ipsilateral gaze palsy due to involvement of the pontine center for lateral gaze, with contralateral hemiplegia.

Millard-Gubler syndrome: ABD and facial nerve palsy with contralateral hemiparesis. This is the pontine counterpart of the Weber syndrome. (The distinction between these two syndromes is very tenuous and will be discussed further in the Motor System.)

The ABD nerve may also be involved in inflammatory disorders, like TBM with basal exudates. In Gradenigo syndrome, there is inflammation of the apex of the petrous temporal bone secondary to severe otitis media and mastoiditis. It is now rarely seen in this era of antibiotics.

The ABD nerve is commonly involved in severe rise of intracranial pressure (ICP) either due to a lesion in the posterior cranial fossa with hydrocephalus or due to idiopathic intracranial hypertension.

THE PUPILS

The easy method of performing the swinging torch light test and analysis of RAPD is already covered in the optic nerve.

The pupil has two basic functions—contraction and dilation, which is performed automatically depending on the ambient light by the parasympathetic and sympathetic innervation, respectively. A few anatomical facts have to be understood in order to explain some of the pupillary abnormalities.

- *Parasympathetic pathway*: The postganglionic fibers originate in the ciliary ganglion within the orbit and innervate the pupillary constrictor muscle of the iris via the short ciliary nerves. Only 3–5% of these fibers innervate the pupillary constrictor muscles. The rest terminate in the ciliary muscle and control accommodation. The importance of this anatomical fact will be discussed when explaining light-near dissociation and the tonic pupil.
- *Sympathetic pathway*: This pathway is very long and initially descends in the brainstem and spinal cord to the level of C8-T1: The first-order preganglionic neurons. They emerge in the base of the neck and then ascend to the superior cervical ganglion: Second-order preganglionic neurons. The third-order neurons arise from the superior cervical ganglion as a plexus around the internal carotid artery (ICA) and ascend with it into the middle cranial fossa and then through the lateral wall of the cavernous sinus and superior orbital fissure to ultimately enter the orbit "piggybacking" with the ophthalmic division of the trigeminal nerve. Thus, lesions of the first-order neurons will have accompanying brainstem and spinal cord signs, second-order neurons may have brachial plexus signs, and third-order neurons may have ICA, cavernous sinus, or superior orbital fissure signs. In clinical practice, the frequency of occurrence of second- and third-order neuronal lesions is more or less equal, comprising 80% of cases. The remaining 20% are lesions affecting the first (central) order neurons.

Anisocoria implies an asymmetry of the pupillary size. When the abnormal pupil is small, there is a lesion of the sympathetic pathways: Horner's syndrome (HS); when the pupil is large, there is involvement of the parasympathetic pathways.

When the Abnormal Pupil is Small

Involvement of the sympathetic pathways—Horner syndrome

Features of Horner Syndrome (HS)

The features of HS are as follows:

- *Pupillary signs*: Ipsilateral miosis and the startle response is either lost or there is a dilatation lag. When a subject is suddenly woken up from deep sleep, there is a reflex dilation of the pupils within 5 seconds because of a sudden increase in sympathetic activity. This is called the startle response which may be lost or the dilation of the pupil may be delayed for over 5 seconds (the dilation lag).
- *Nonpupillary signs*: There is a subtle ptosis because of weakness of Mueller's muscle, conjunctival congestion because of paresis of the vasomotor fibers, and anhidrosis because of paresis of the sudomotor fibers.

Lesions Producing Horner Syndrome

Lesions producing Horner Syndrome are as follows:

- *Involvement of the central pathways*: The most common lesions encountered in clinical practice are Wallenberg syndrome (posterior inferior cerebellar artery infarct), syringomyelia, and inflammatory myelitis.
- *Involvement of the preganglionic second-order neurons*: The most common etiology is due to a Pancoast tumor or metastasis from breast cancer. Besides involving the sympathetic pathways as they emerge from the C8-T1 segments of the spinal cord, they also involve the upper roots of the brachial plexus. Hence, occult malignancy should be considered in any patient with a nontraumatic new-onset HS and shoulder/arm pain and wasting of the distal part of the ipsilateral upper limb, particularly if the patient is an adult male and a heavy smoker.
- *Involvement of the postganglionic third-order neurons*: In this involvement, the clinical relevance is of spontaneous or traumatic ICA dissection. It presents with unilateral head and/or anterior neck pain, focal cerebral ischemic features, and HS. It should be stressed that in this lesion, the anhidrosis is absent or restricted to the distribution of the first division of the trigeminal nerve as the sudomotor fibers "piggyback" with the ophthalmic division of the trigeminal nerve while entering the orbit. The rest of the face is spared because the sudomotor fibers from the superior cervical ganglia travel along the external carotid artery which is not involved in the dissection. This pattern of anhidrosis is practically indicative of a postganglionic third-order neuronal lesion.

It is well recognized that in HS, the temperature of the skin rises together with conjunctival congestion because of loss of vasomotor control. One other observation that I have made over the years but never studied scientifically is the dryness of the skin, particularly in patients with oily skins. As the sudomotor fibers also innervate the sebaceous glands, together with anhidrosis, the skin is dry in comparison to the oily skin in the contiguous area on the normal side. This needs confirmation and I hope some young dynamic neurologist takes up this task.

When the Abnormal Pupil is Dilated

Involvement of the parasympathetic pathways.

The first clinical tip that I can give you is that the pupil is dilated irrespective of the fact whether the lesion is pre- or postganglionic. Clinically, most of the lesions are preganglionic due to involvement of the OCM nerve. A lot of stress has been put on OCM nerve palsies with and without pupillary involvement. In this context, the following points should be remembered:

- OCM nerve palsy with or without pupillary involvement applies only to partial OCM nerve palsy, as in total palsy the pupil is fully dilated.
- OCM nerve palsy with or without pupillary involvement contributes nothing to the differential diagnosis or etiology. However, a general

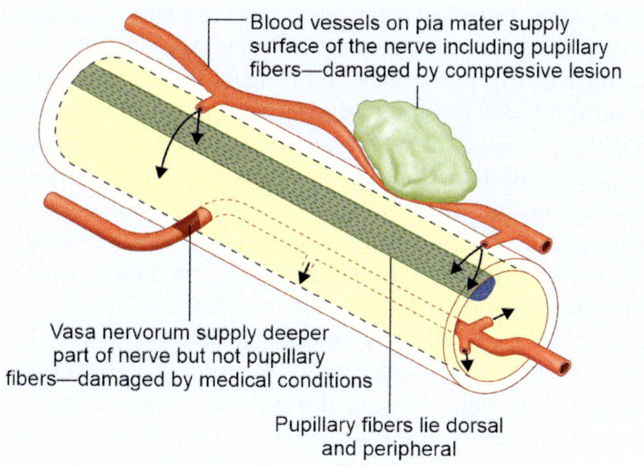

FIG. 6.5: Oculomotor nerve showing the lay of the pupillary and fibers to the external ocular muscles.

Courtesy: Professor Vivek Lal, PGIMER, Chandigarh.

"rule of the thumb" is that OCM nerve palsy with pupillary involvement is usually due to compression, whereas OCM nerve palsy with pupillary sparing is usually due to metabolic causes. This is because the pupillary fibers travel superficially in the OCM nerve, whereas fibers to the external ocular muscles are deep within the nerve **(Fig. 6.5)**.

- As with any rule of the thumb, there are exceptions to the rule. Pupil-sparing OCM nerve palsy occurs in the early stages of compressive pathology. Therefore, a close follow-up is required to monitor pupillary involvement. Thus, any patient with a progressive external ophthalmoplegia warrants neuroimaging as a compressive cause is very likely. Conversely, diabetic OCM nerve palsy is the most common cause of metabolic involvement, but only 50% have pupillary sparing.

POSTGANGLIONIC OCULOMOTOR NERVE PALSY

In postganglionic involvement, the lesion is in the ciliary ganglion or short ciliary nerves within the orbit or the eye itself. Clinically, the following features are observed. In the acute stage, the pupil is large, round, and nonreactive to direct and consensual light reflex. Later, the pupil constricts, reversing anisocoria, and has an irregular shape. The light reflex is attenuated or absent. In contrast, the pupil shows an exaggerated miosis to accommodative efforts. This is called the "light-near dissociation." In addition, the miotic pupil takes a long time to dilate when vision shifts to a distant object—the tonic pupil.

The light-near dissociation and the tonic pupil are based on anatomical facts. As mentioned earlier, 95–97% of the fibers from the ciliary ganglion innervate the ciliary muscles. After a lesion of the ciliary ganglion or short ciliary nerves, these "accommodation" fibers reinnervate the pupillary constrictor muscle. This gives rise to an exaggerated miotic response of the pupil to accommodation but not to the light reflex. Secondly, the pupil takes a prolonged time to dilation when accommodation is over. Thus, a tonic pupil with light-near dissociation is pathognomonic of a postganglionic parasympathetic lesion. The etiologies are varied; unilateral lesions are trauma, inflammatory, neoplastic, or idiopathic—the Holmes–Adie syndrome. Bilateral lesions are usually due to pure autonomic failure associated with Sjögren or paraneoplastic syndromes and rarely in amyloidosis.

Lastly, in an entity of the past, similar involvement was described in tertiary syphilis as the Argyll–Robertson (AR) pupil. The AR pupils are usually small and irregular in shape. Despite the small size, there is light-near dissociation. The exact site of the lesion is not known but is believed to be ventral to the aqueduct in the upper midbrain involving the pretectal nuclear connections. Pseudo-AR pupils may be seen in diabetes and neurosarcoidosis.

A CLINICAL APPROACH TO OPHTHALMOPLEGIAS

Visual performance is best when the image of the target is held steady on the fovea. There are six oculomotor systems which perform this task.

The fixation system holds the eyes steady on the target during intense gaze.

Three systems keep the visual target in the environment on the fovea: The pursuit (slow), the saccadic (fast), and the vergence systems. The latter is the only supranuclear system which produces dysconjugate eye movements. Two systems stabilize the eyes during head movement: The oculovestibular reflex (OVR) and the optokinetic system. Thus, our eye movements are controlled by the coordinated functioning of these six systems. In turn, these systems function at five different levels of the nervous system: Supranuclear, internuclear, nuclear/infranuclear level, at the level of the myoneural junction, and the extrinsic ocular muscle. Hence, ophthalmoplegias occur at these five different levels.

Supranuclear Ophthalmoplegia

- Since the supranuclear pathways are involved in conjugate eye movements, lesions of these pathways produce conjugate gaze palsies. This may involve fast (saccadic) or slow (pursuit) eye movements or both. Selective saccadic eye movement involvement is easily detected by the absence of optokinetic nystagmus.
- The patient does not complain of diplopia and on inspection of the eyes, in the primary position, there is no squint. There are two exceptions to this statement. Skew deviation in which the pupil on the affected side is higher than the opposite side one, i.e., dysconjugate in the vertical axis.

Supranuclear skew deviation is usually seen in lesions of the thalamus, brainstem, or cerebellum. In such cases, in addition to the skew deviation of the eyes, there will be symptoms and signs of thalamic, brainstem, or cerebellar involvement. Note that the most common cause of skew deviation is usually due to SO palsy. The second exception is Perinaud dorsal midbrain syndrome. The lesion involves the tectal area of the midbrain and the clinical features are supranuclear vertical gaze palsy, upward more than downward, lid retraction on attempted upward gaze, convergence-retraction nystagmus, pupillary light-near dissociation, and pseudo-abduction deficit caused by excessive convergence tone—dysconjugate eyes.

The etiologies of supranuclear ophthalmoplegias are strokes, tumors involving the midbrain, and neurodegenerative diseases. In day-to-day practice, the most common form of supranuclear gaze palsy is seen in acute strokes **(Figs. 6.6A and B)**. In a hemispheric lesion, there is a paralytic involvement of the cortical eye fields resulting in an overaction of the contralateral intact eye fields. This results in a conjugate deviation of the eyes to the side of the lesion. In a pontine lesion, there is an ipsilateral paralysis of the center for lateral gaze, with a contralateral conjugate deviation, i.e., the eyes look toward the hemiplegic side.

The other commonly seen supranuclear ophthalmoplegias in India are the vertical gaze palsy of progressive supranuclear palsy (PSP) and the slow

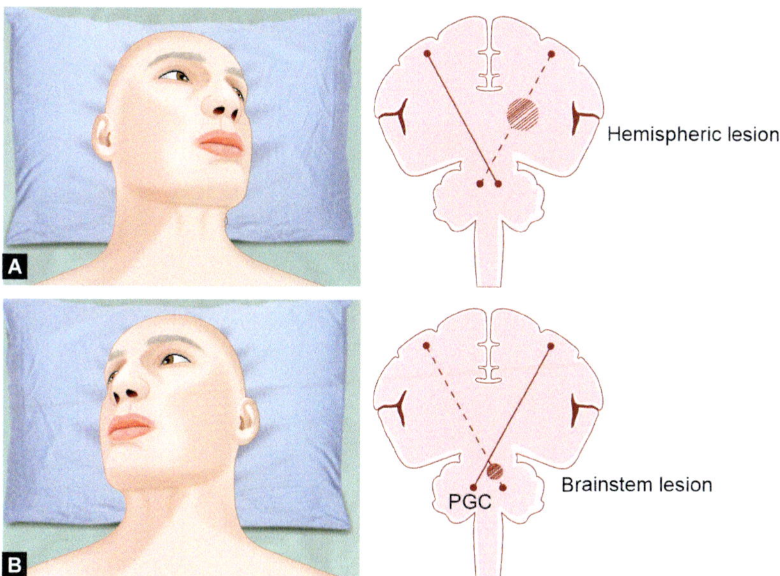

FIGS. 6.6A AND B: Conjugate gaze deviation in acute strokes.
(PGC: pontine gaze centre)

eye movements of spinocerebellar ataxia type 2 (SCA2). Slow saccades may also be seen in Parkinson's and Huntington's disease.

Internuclear Ophthalmoplegias

In internuclear ophthalmoplegias (INO), the lesion is in the medial longitudinal fasciculus (MLF) which connects the ABD nerve nucleus (LR) in the pons to the appropriate part of the contralateral OCM nerve (MR) nucleus in the midbrain (see Fig. 9.1 on page 65). This implies that an INO is invariably due to an intrinsic brainstem lesion. In an INO, the eyes are conjugate in the primary position. On lateral gaze, away from the side of the lesion, there is complete abduction (LR action), but the adduction of the contralateral eye (MR action) is weak or absent as the MR does not get any signals due to the MLF lesion. Thus, the eyes become dysconjugate on lateral gaze with the possibility of diplopia. But the main feature of INO is nystagmus in the abducting eye. The physiological mechanism of this is as follows:

Say the patient has a right MLF lesion. Thus, there is no adduction of the right eye. Nature tries to adduct the right eye by recruiting convergence, whose pathways are in the rostral part of the midbrain. With this recruitment, the right eye adducts but so does the left eye. The image of the target moves away from the fovea of the left eye. Therefore, there is a correcting saccade. This sequence of events is repeated, generating an abducting nystagmus. INO is most commonly seen in strokes and multiple sclerosis (MS) **(Fig. 6.7)**. The other less common conditions are brainstem encephalitis, traumatic brain injury (TBI), and rarely in the early stages of a brainstem glioma.

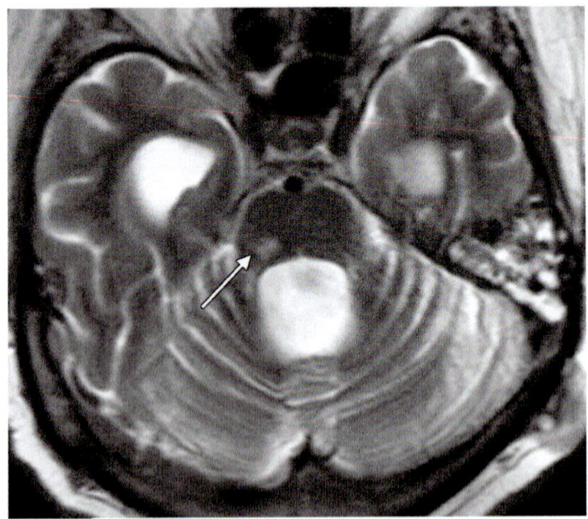

FIG. 6.7: T2W MRI showing a plaque of MS involving the right MLF (arrow).
(MLF: medial longitudinal fasciculus; MRI: magnetic resonance imaging; MS: multiple sclerosis; T2W: T2-weighted)

Nuclear and Infranuclear Ophthalmoplegias

This is already covered earlier in this chapter. Here, I would like to mention about Wernicke encephalopathy (WE). This results from thiamine deficiency due to malnutrition, malabsorption, or increased metabolic demands usually in alcoholics and malnourished individuals. It has a triad of confusion, ophthalmoplegias, and ataxia. Confusion and ophthalmoplegias occur in 90–96% of cases, whereas ataxia is less common. It must be noted that there is a spectrum of ophthalmoplegias in WE. The most common form of ophthalmoplegia is a gaze paretic nystagmus (87%) followed by LR palsy, conjugate gaze palsy, and even total external ophthalmoplegia. If untreated, it can progress over days or weeks to coma or even death. The importance of recognizing this entity is the rapid improvement of all symptoms with IV thiamine, an amenable and gratifyingly treatable condition. The MRI will show symmetrical hyperintense signals in the medial thalamus, floor of the OCM ventricle, mammillary bodies, and periaqueductal gray matter **(Figs. 6.8A and B)**.

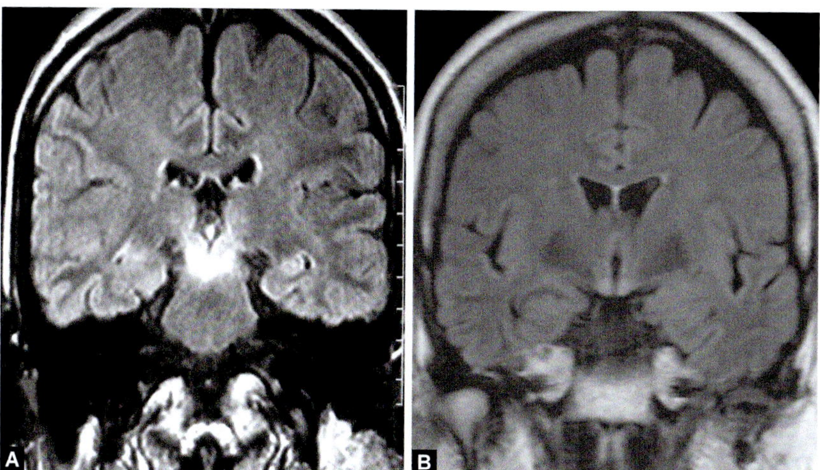

FIGS. 6.8A AND B: Wernicke encephalopathy. FLAIR coronal images showing (A) hyperintense signals in the thalamus and floor of the III ventricle and (B) hyperintense signals in the mammillary bodies.

(FLAIR: fluid attenuated inversion recovery)

Myoneural Junction and Myopathic Ophthalmoplegias

The classic myoneural junction (MNJ) ophthalmoplegia is ocular MG. The hallmark of the ophthalmoplegia and ptosis in MG is fluctuation, particularly in the ptosis. The latter can be rapidly improved by cooling the supraorbital area with an ice cube. Botulinum toxin-induced ophthalmoplegias and ptosis can mimic MG **(Figs. 6.9A to C)**. However, in the acute phase of the toxicity, the involvement is bilateral, symmetrical, very severe, and fixed (no fluctuation). In ocular and mitochondrial myopathies with progressive

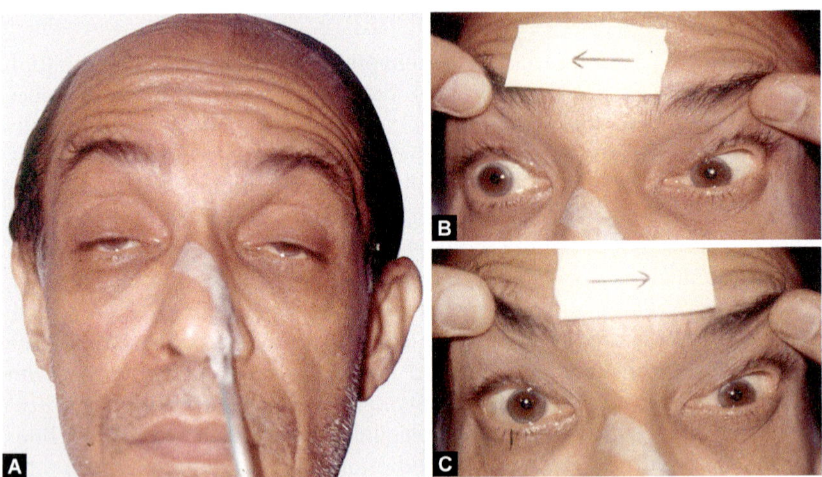

FIGS. 6.9A TO C: Patient has acute botulinum toxicity. Note severe bilateral ptosis and total external ophthalmoplegia. The patient also had dysphagia which required Ryles tube feeding.

external ophthalmoplegia, the involvement is bilateral and symmetrical. Hence, the patients do not complain of diplopia.

Table 6.2 shows the clinical differentiation of the various levels of ophthalmoplegias.

TABLE 6.2: Clinical differentiation of ophthalmoplegias.

Site	Diplopia	Primary position	Pupil	Long tracts
Supranuclear	Nil	N	N	Yes
Internuclear	Yes	N but abnormal in lateral gaze	N	Yes
Nuclear	Yes	Squint	+/–	Yes
Infranuclear	Yes	Squint	+/–	No
MN junction	Yes	Squint	N	No
Myopathies	No	N but with ptosis	N	No

(N: normal; +/–: maybe; MN: myoneural)

RECOMMENDED ARTICLES

1. Dinkin M. Diagnostic approach to diplopia. Continuum-Neuro-Ophthalmol. 2014;20:942-65.
2. Katrak SM, Irani AM. An approach to pupillary disorders- physiology and pathology. In: Vivek Lal (Ed). A Clinical Approach to Neuro-Ophthalmic Disorders, 1st edition. Florida: CBS Press; 2022. Pp. 158-62.
3. Kung NH, Van Stavern GP. Isolated ocular motor palsies. Semin Neurol. 2015;35:539-48.
4. Walsh TJ (Ed). Diplopia. In: TJ Walsh (Ed). Neuro-Ophthalmology: Clinical Signs and Symptoms. Philadelphia: Lea & Febiger; 1978. pp. 61-91.

CHAPTER 7

Cranial Nerve 5: The Trigeminal Nerve

The trigeminal nerve is a predominantly sensory nerve with a small motor component. It innervates the face, the teeth and oral cavity, the nasal mucosa, the anterior half of the scalp, the dura mater, and the intracranial vasculature. It also provides proprioception from the muscles of mastication and the face. The motor component emerges as a small motor root, which soon merges with the mandibular division of the nerve and innervates the muscles of mastication.

The sensory component consists of three divisions: (1) The ophthalmic (V-1), (2) the maxillary (V-2), and (3) the mandibular (V-3) divisions, which end in the Gasserian ganglion (GasG). Before terminating in the GasG, V-1 is dorsal, V-2 is in the middle, and V-3 is ventral. Subsequent to the GasG the anatomy is reversed, i.e., the V-1 is ventral and the V-3 is dorsal.

Within the pons the course of these fibers is rather complex. Fibers for pain/temperature enter the spinal tract and descend to various levels; the V-1 fibers do not descend as far as the V-2 and V-3 fibers. They then synapse with the neighboring nuclei of the spinal tract. The second order neurons crossover and ascend as the ventral trigeminothalamic tract (TTT) enroute to the ventroposterior medial (VPM) nucleus of the thalamus. The somatotropic organization of the fibers from the three divisions in the spinal tract is responsible for the "onion peel" pattern of sensory impairment, i.e., concentric circles of sensory impairment starting from the perioral area and spreading to the preauricular area. Thus, this pattern is suggestive of a lesion of the trigeminal sensory tract from the mid-pons to the high cervical cord. This pattern is commonly seen in syringomyelia/bulbia. Sensory loss in the classical distribution suggests involvement of any of the three divisions up to the GasG.

Fibers subserving light touch and proprioception predominantly terminate in the principal sensory nucleus in the rostral pons. The second order neurons then crossover and ascend in the ventral TTT to end in the VPM nucleus of the thalamus.

The mesencephalic nucleus in the rostral pons mainly receives proprioceptive impulses from the masticatory muscles. It also has a collateral connection with the neurons in the neighboring reticular formation. Thus, when you ask an individual to clench his jaw, the sluggish deep tendon reflex (DTR) is easily elicited because of an increase in reticulospinal tone to the intrafusal fibers of the muscle spindle.

The motor component consists of bilateral cortical innervations of the motor nucleus in the rostral pons. The motor root emerges from the ventrolateral aspect of the pons, runs along the inferior surface of the GasG and merges into V-3 division of the nerve. It supplies the four primary muscles of mastication: (1) Masseter, (2) temporalis, (3) medial, and (4) lateral pterygoids. The lateral pterygoid is the main muscle which opens the mouth. In unilateral paralysis, the normal lateral pterygoid is responsible for the lateral deviation of the jaw to the paralyzed side.

A lot has been written about the trigeminal nerve in the books of neurological examination. Here, I would like to stress on a few points in the sensory testing of the nerve and motor weakness.

Sensory testing: Eliciting a corneal reflex (CR) properly is an art. Very often resident doctors approach the patient from the front; the patient blinks frequently, and therefore, the doctor touches the sclera instead of the cornea. The easy practical way to elicit the CR is to form a good wisp of cotton wool beforehand, if necessary wet your fingers in order to do this. Stand on one side of the patient and hold the wisp of cotton in your left hand while testing the right CR and vice versa for the left eye. Ask the patient to look up and away from the side being tested. The upper eyelid is thus elevated, and the cornea is properly exposed. Then touch the upper part of the cornea quickly. When the CR is preserved, bilateral blinking is observed.

In cases of acoustic neuromas, there may be associated facial weakness with weak or absent blinking. Under these circumstances the integrity of the CR is judged by tearing ipsilaterally (in partial facial nerve involvement) or contralateral blinking. The absence of the CR together with dense facial weakness, as seen commonly in acoustic neuroma, is a dangerous combination leading to exposure keratitis. In such cases I have requested my ophthalmic colleagues to perform a lateral tarsorrhaphy to protect the eye. Similarly in patients who are comatose or with Guillain-Barré syndrome (GBS) and bilateral facial palsy, I have advised a similar procedure.

When testing pain in the ophthalmic division of the trigeminal nerve, it is always a good practice to go beyond the intermeatal line (a line drawn from one external auditory meatus to the other) over the vertex of the scalp. The area posterior to the intermeatal line is supplied by the C2 spinal root. If there is impairment of pain in the ophthalmic division, the patient will appreciate the sudden increase in pain when you go posterior to the intermeatal line, thus confirming impairment of pain in the ophthalmic division.

Similarly, perioral pain sensations must be compared to the posterior part of the face, to exclude the "onion peel" pattern, which is suggestive of involvement of the sensory tract in the mid-pons (rostral tract) and spinal cord (caudal tract).

In a stuporous/comatose patient, one frequently has to give a prognosis about the outcome. Therefore, one should always give a supraorbital painful stimulus and observe for grimacing. If the patient grimaces, the prognosis is always better than the absence of grimacing. The afferent part of this reflex arc is via the ophthalmic division and the TTT and the efferent limb is via the corticobulbar tracts up to the facial nucleus in the pons. Thus, this circuit is purely within the brainstem and a good prognostic parameter. Secondly, grimacing is more voluntary than reflex motor activity, reflecting a better level of consciousness. Lastly, while assessing for brain death, one should always test the response to deep supraorbital painful stimulus as the pathways are purely restricted to the brainstem. At times, deep painful stimuli over the limbs may produce some movements which are purely of spinal cord reflex origin.

It is said that proprioception cannot be adequately tested in the trigeminal distribution. Beyond the concha, the greater part of the pinna of the ear is supplied by the auriculotemporal nerve, which originates from the mandibular division of the trigeminal nerve and the lesser occipital nerve (C2-3). Therefore, one can test proprioception in the joint distribution of the mandibular division and C2-3 by moving the pinna of the ear forward or backward. I have used this method in the rare cases of syringobulbia, to test proprioception over the face.

Motor weakness in the muscles innervated by the trigeminal nerve: Isolated pure motor trigeminal weakness is a rarity. It is well recognized that this entity is seen together with wasting in the late stages of motor neuron disease. It is also seen in severe myasthenia gravis (MG) but without wasting. In the latter, there may be a "jaw drop." A less well-recognized fact is that poliomyelitis can produce acute weakness and wasting of the temporalis and masseter muscles particularly in the pediatric age group. This fortunately is a thing of the past. The last time I saw a crop of such cases was in 1981 during the second epidemic of EV-70 disease—a polioclastic illness. Again, it is well recognized that those muscles that are well exercised in the preparalytic phase of a polioclastic disease, like EV-70, are maximally involved. It is interesting to note that in the majority of these cases, which I saw in 1981, had the habit of chewing pan or betel nut.

CHAPTER 8

Cranial Nerve 7: The Facial Nerve

The facial nerve is mainly a motor nerve—the main motor trunk and the nerve to the stapedius—but has a sensory and parasympathetic component through the nervus intermedius (NI). The motor component innervates the facial muscles for voluntary and emotional facial expressions. The sensory component conveys taste from the anterior two-thirds of the tongue and the parasympathetic component innervates the salivary and lacrimal glands and the mucosa of the nose and oral cavity.

Facial expressions from a central lesion have two components: (1) Voluntary facial expressions and (2) spontaneous emotional facial expressions.

1. *Voluntary facial expressions*: The supranuclear pathways arise from the motor cortex, ventrolateral supplementary motor area, and the premotor cortex. This pathway then descends as the corticobulbar tract ipsilaterally up to the rostral pons and then crosses over to the opposite side to innervate the facial nucleus in the caudal pons. The upper face has bilateral innervation, whereas the lower face has only unilateral.

   Based on these anatomical facts, the clinical implications are: Lesions up to the rostral pons produce a contralateral hemiplegia with upper motor neuron (UMN) facial palsy (a standard hemiplegia). Lesions in the caudal pons produce an ipsilateral facial palsy with contralateral hemiplegia. A rare anatomical variation is that the upper face may have a unilateral innervation. In my 50 years of clinical practice, I saw only one patient with acute onset of what looked like a left lower motor neuron (LMN) facial palsy with an ipsilateral hemiplegia. He also had conjugate gaze deviation to the right. Neuroimaging showed an infarct in the centrum semiovale.

   Cortical lesions usually produce an UMN facial palsy, which is associated with the paresis of the ipsilateral tongue because of the proximity of the cortical representation of the tongue and face. A loss of ability to wink one eye is a sensitive test of early corticopontine tract involvement and may be noted even when bilateral blinking is intact.
2. *Emotional facial expressions*: The supranuclear pathways arise from the contralateral cingulate gyrus with inputs from the limbic system,

striatum, globus pallidus, thalamus, and hypothalamus. Emotional control tracts do not descend in the internal capsule together with the corticobulbar tracts but descend as a separate cortically originating extrapyramidal system. The clinical implications are as follows: As the supranuclear control of voluntary and emotional facial expressions has separate centers and pathways, there can be a dissociation of voluntary and emotional movements. A commonly seen phenomenon is paralysis of voluntary facial expression with preservation of emotional movements in a hemiplegic patient. Rarely, with lesions in the ventrolateral thalamus, globus pallidus, or hypothalamus, the converse can occur, i.e., "emotional" palsy without "voluntary" palsy.

Based on **Figure 8.1**, the various levels of involvement of the facial nerve together with the clinical findings are as follows:

1. The lesion is distal to the branching of the chorda tympani. The clinical features are LMN paralysis of the facial nerve alone. If the nerve is involved distal to the stylomastoid foramen (SMF), some of the branches of the facial nerve may escape producing patchy involvement of the facial muscles. If the facial nerve is involved at the SMF, the paralysis of the facial muscles is severe together with pain behind the ear—the characteristic features of a Bell's palsy.
2. The lesion is in the facial canal between the nerve to the stapedius and chorda tympani. The clinical features are LMN facial paralysis together with loss of taste in the anterior two-thirds of the tongue + impairment of salivary secretions.

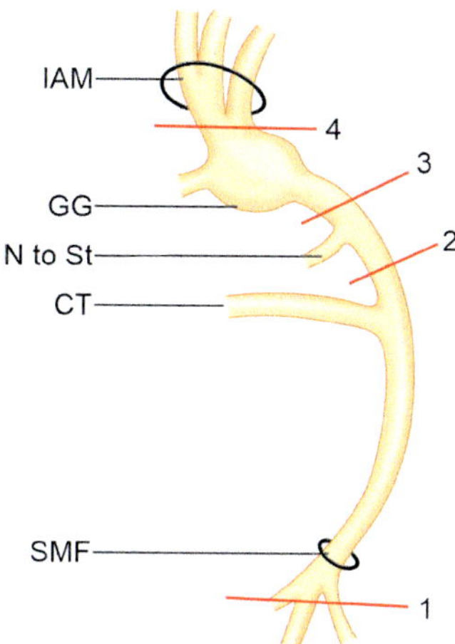

FIG. 8.1: Levels of involvement of the peripheral part of the facial nerve (see text for more details).

(CT: chorda tympani; GG: geniculate ganglion; IAM: internal auditory meatus; N to St: nerve to stapedius; SMF: stylomastoid foramen)

3. The lesion is between the nerve to the stapedius and the geniculate ganglion (GG). The clinical features are the same as in number 2, but in addition, there is hyperacusis because of the involvement of the nerve to the stapedius.
4. The lesion is in between the internal auditory meatus (IAM) and the GG. The clinical features are a combination of 2 and 3, i.e., facial paralysis, loss of taste, impaired salivary secretions, and hyperacusis. In addition, there may be sensory neural deafness if the acoustic nerve is involved. In the latter event, hyperacusis is absent.

The facial nerve may also be involved intracranially in basal lesions. The clinical features will be similar to 4, but in addition, other basal cranial nerves may be involved, such as acoustic, abducens, glossopharyngeal, vagus, or hypoglossal. Lastly, nuclear lesions within the pons produce LMN facial involvement with long tract signs—Millard-Gubler syndrome, ipsilateral 7th nerve palsy with contralateral hemiplegia. Because of the peculiar anatomical relationship of the intraparenchymatous part of the facial nerve with the abducens nucleus, the lateral rectus is practically always involved. Since the medial part of the abducens nucleus serves as the pontine center for lateral gaze, the Foville syndrome involves ipsilateral 7th nerve with lateral rectus/ lateral gaze palsy with contralateral hemiplegia.

Hence, in a case of LMN facial palsy, ask the following questions:

Is there a change in taste in the anterior two-thirds of the tongue? If so, the facial nerve is involved in the mastoid segment distally.

Do you have any problem in hearing? If the answer is yes and there is hyperacusis, there is involvement of the nerve to the stapedius as well. If the patient complains of deafness in the ipsilateral ear, the involvement is at the level of the IAM. Note that for all practical purposes, involvement of the facial nerve in the mastoid segment will produce hyperacusis and impaired taste in the anterior two-thirds of the tongue.

Do you have pain behind the ear? If the answer is yes, the facial palsy is due to involvement of the nerve at or just beyond the SMF.

Is your affected eye dry? Decreased tearing with deep pain in the region of the ear is suggestive of lesions of the GG. This usually occurs with herpes zoster infection—the Ramsay-Hunt syndrome.

TIPS DURING EXAMINATION OF THE FACIAL NERVE

During examination, look for symmetry of blinking. In partial weakness of the orbicularis oculi, incomplete closure of the affected eye may occur without altering the rate of blinking. With the glabellar tap, normally, both eyes blink simultaneously. With very early facial palsy, on glabellar tap, the ipsilateral blink is not only reduced in strength but slightly delayed compared to the normal side. This may be the earliest sign of ensuing facial palsy. Lastly, when a lesion of the 7th nerve is in doubt, ask the patient to close his eyes tightly and then the examiner tries to open the upper eyelid by exerting an upward pressure with his thumb. In this way, the motor strength of the

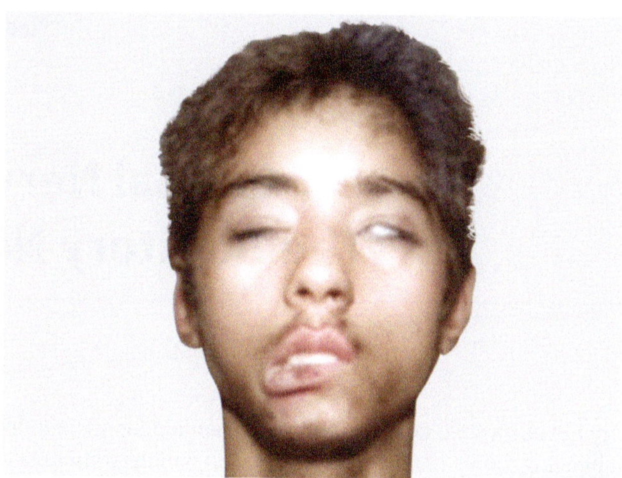

FIG. 8.2: Bilateral facial paresis in Madras motor neuron disease (MND).

orbicularis oculi can be compared, and early weakness may be detected. Also, during an attempt to open the eyelid, the amplitude and rate of upper lid vibration are reduced.

Synkinesis vs. hemifacial spasm (HFS): Facial synkinesis occurs after a facial nerve palsy because of aberrant regeneration. HFS arises de novo because of an ectatic loop of the anterior inferior cerebellar artery (AICA) compressing the facial nerve. HFS develops in older patients and is twice as common in women than men. The twitching usually begins in the orbicularis oculi and may be difficult to differentiate from facial synkinesis. The easiest way to differentiate one from the other is to ask the patient to blink three times. In facial synkinesis, there is a simultaneous twitch of the orbicularis oris on the affected side. Then ask the patient to purse her/his lips tightly. There is a simultaneous narrowing of the affected palpebral fissure—what I call the "Lalita Pawar" sign, after the late actress of yesterday years who, I believe, had facial synkinesis.

Prognosis in Bell's palsy: The prognosis for recovery in Bell's palsy is always good. The vast majority of patients recover whether treated with steroids or not. However, the prognosis for recovery in the Ramsay-Hunt syndrome (involvement of the facial nerve due to herpes zoster) is poor, particularly if there is a lack of tearing in the affected eye suggestive of involvement of the GG. Hence, look closely for herpetic scabs in or around the external auditory meatus. Lastly, an isolated acute LMN facial palsy in children or young adults can be due to a polioclastic illness, i.e., polio or EV-70 disease. If the palsy is insidious, it is seen in the early stages of Madras motor neuron disease (MND) **(Fig. 8.2)**.

In recent times, loss of taste, ageusia, has gained importance as an early sign of COVID-19 infection.

CHAPTER 9

Cranial Nerve 8: The Auditory Nerve

The auditory nerve has two components: (1) Cochlear/acoustic nerve, which subserves hearing, and (2) vestibular nerve, which transmits impulses concerned with orientation of the body in space. Although these two components are functionally separate, they are united by a common trunk which passes centrally through the internal auditory meatus (IAM) in company with the facial nerve and the nervus intermedius. After traversing the region of the cerebellopontine angle (CPA), the auditory nerve enters the caudal part of the pons and then the two components run separate courses. The complex bilateral courses through the brainstem up to the cortical centers are beyond the scope of this book.

COCHLEAR/ACOUSTIC NERVE: CLINICAL EXAMINATION FOR HEARING

This is usually done by utilizing 128 (low-frequency), 256 (mid-frequency), and 512 (high-frequency) tuning forks. The tuning fork is tapped and placed next to the tragus of the ear for air conduction (AC) and on the mastoid bone for bone conduction (BC). The drawback of this method is that the intensity of the sounds (tapping of the tuning fork) is difficult to standardize for both sides. Nevertheless, this localizes impaired acuity of hearing (A/H) well.

Normally, AC is better than BC. In local disorders of the ear, BC > AC—conductive deafness (CD) and in sensorineural deafness (SND) both are impaired, but AC is always more impaired than BC until there is total deafness.

Textbooks mention the whispering test at various distances to judge A/H. What I find very convenient is to crinkle the patient's hair and compare the two sides. This ensures that the intensity of the sound and the distance are similar in both ears. The limitations of this method are in males who are bald or with totally shaven heads as is the trend nowadays. Lastly, if you want to be extremely meticulous, put one earpiece of a stethoscope in one ear, tap a 512-Hz tuning fork extremely lightly, and place it on the diaphragm of the stethoscope. Time the vibration sound in that ear and then repeat the process for comparison in the other ear. Although the distance from the diaphragm to the ear is the same, the intensity of the sound may differ reducing the sensitivity of this test. But if there is an inequality of the sound in one ear, then this is a sensitive way of picking up early impairment of hearing. Unfortunately, in modern stethoscopes, one is not able to pinch the tubing to either ear as was possible in the older versions of stethoscopes. This would ensure that the intensity and the distance are similar for both ears. Having mentioned this method, I confess that I have rarely used it, as clinically, the other methods are good enough to lateralize impairment of hearing.

As a general rule, CD is produced by local causes in the external or middle ear. On the other hand, SND can be peripheral (inner ear and extracranial) or central (intracranial) but extramedullary usually in the CPA. Central deafness due to lesions of the central pathway is very rare due to bilaterality of the auditory system. In routine clinical practice, lesions of the central pathways do not cause any detectable deficits and for all practical purposes should not be considered as a cause of deafness.

Rinne's and Weber's tests are usually used for conductive hearing loss. In a patient who gives totally unreliable answers on sensory testing in the limbs, I have used Weber's test to judge his/her reliability. In CD, when you close one ear (say the right), during Weber's test, the patient will lateralize to the right ear. An unreliable patient feels that the doctor has closed my right ear and wants me to point to the left ear and that is exactly what he/she does indicating their unreliability.

TINNITUS

An irritative lesion of the labyrinth or cochlear nerve manifests as subjective noises: Roaring, humming, whistling, or hissing. In the middle ear, only otosclerosis deserves mention. It is a disorder of the cochlear hair or ganglion cells. The tinnitus is constant in comparison to that with SND where the intensity varies. Tinnitus can become particularly intense in otosclerosis when the internal ear is involved, and this is associated with impaired A/H. Tinnitus with vertigo suggests involvement of the neighboring vestibular nerve. Later on, the neighboring 7th nerve may also be affected.

Tinnitus with symptoms and signs of medullary, pons, or cerebellar involvement indicates an intracranial irritative lesion. By far, the most common pathology is an acoustic neuroma in which tinnitus is usually the initial symptom. Vertigo occurs in a small percentage but almost invariably, all patients become deaf at which stage tinnitus disappears. Therefore, tinnitus that is unilateral, fluctuating in intensity, and later associated with deafness is indicative of a serious underlying condition and warrants magnetic resonance imaging (MRI) of the brain.

Meniere's disease (MD) also produces tinnitus, but the main symptom is paroxysmal vertigo followed by deafness. Occasionally, this entity is mistakenly diagnosed as vestibular neuronitis. The absence of tinnitus and impaired hearing help distinguish vestibular neuronitis from MD.

The vestibular nerve gets inputs from five structures: The utricle, the saccule, and the three semicircular canals (SCC). The main symptom is vertigo. Besides the true spinning sensation, the lay person may include a host of nonspecific symptoms into the common word such as "giddiness," "dizziness," "chakkar," or "vertigo." As I often tell my students, the symptom of "chakkar" is likely to put the examiner into a spin or "chakkar" of his own. Not infrequently, the patient has seen an ophthalmologist, ear-nose-throat (ENT) surgeon, and a physician before landing up with the neurologist—"the doctor ka chakkar" as I call it. This phenomenon is worldwide, and Professor W Bryan Matthews succinctly mentioned in his monogram, Practical Neurology, 2nd edition, 1970, "there can be few physicians so dedicated to their art, that they do not experience a slight decline in spirits on learning that their patient's complaint is of giddiness".

A BRIEF PRACTICAL ANATOMY AND PHYSIOLOGY OF THE VESTIBULAR SYSTEM

Only a few relevant points of the vestibular system will be outlined here:

- The vestibular system should be considered as a paired system—, one on either side, and the brain is constantly comparing the functions of the two sides.
- Together, the three SCCs and the physiologically distinct otolith organs (utricle and saccule) perform three distinct functions.
    - *Detection of head position vis-à-vis the body and gravity*: This is performed by the otolith organs.
    - *Detection of head motion*: Angular acceleration by the SCCs and linear acceleration by the otolith systems
    - *Control of the vestibule-ocular response (VOR):* This is also known as the doll's eye maneuver. There is an automatic compensation of any head movement with an equal and opposite eye movement to keep the image of the object on the fovea. Simply put, the VOR maintains clear vision during head movement.

Physiology of the horizontal VOR ***(Fig. 9.1)***: When the head turns to the right, there is an excitatory stimulation of the horizontal SCC. These excitatory impulses travel via the auditory nerve to the medial vestibular nucleus which transmits excitatory impulses to the interneurons in the opposite abducens nucleus. From here, the impulses travel to the motor neurons of the left lateral rectus and via the MLF to the appropriate part of the oculomotor nucleus in the midbrain which subserves the right medial rectus. This results

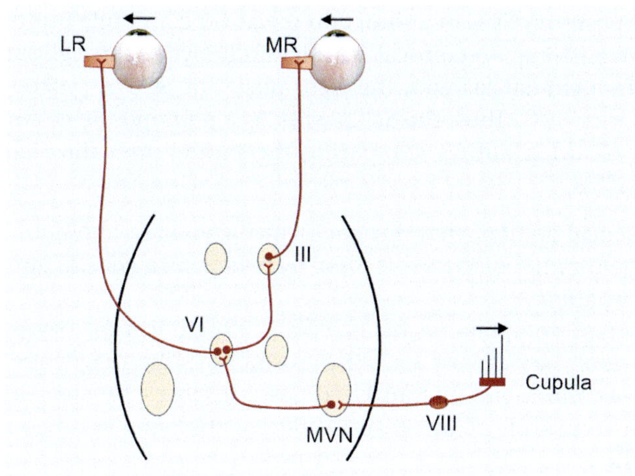

FIG. 9.1: Vestibulo-ocular reflex.

(LR: lateral rectus; MR: medial rectus; MVN: medial vestibular nucleus; III, VI: cranial nuclei; VIII: auditory nerve)

The line connecting VI to III represents the medial longitudinal fasciculus (MLF).

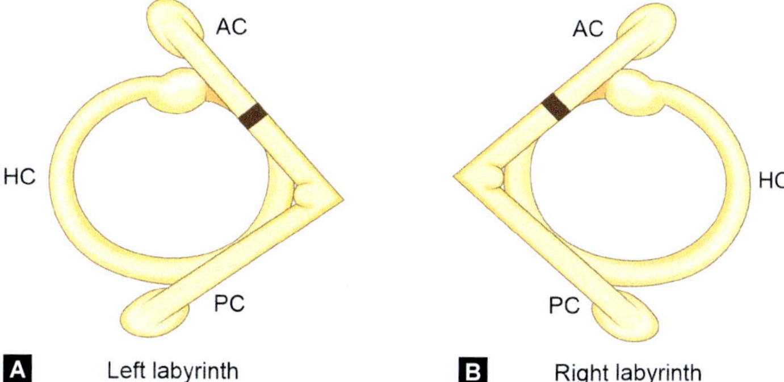

FIGS. 9.2A AND B: Orientation of the semicircular canals. Note that (A) AC/PC are parallel to (B) PC/AC and work in tandem.

(AC: anterior semicircular canals; HC: horizontal semicircular canals; PC: posterior semicircular canals)

in a conjugate gaze deviation to the left. Hence, when the head turns to the right, the eyes move to the left and vice versa—the so-called doll's eye or oculocephalic maneuver.

- A unique feature of the vestibular physiology is the pairing of the vestibular organs **(Figs. 9.2A and B)**. The left anterior SCC is parallel with the right posterior SCC. Bending the head to the right will stimulate the right anterior SCC in a direction away from the ampulla (ampullofugal) and the left posterior SCC in a direction toward the ampulla (ampullopetal), thus establishing a reciprocal interaction between the right and the left SCCs. In a similar fashion, the right posterior SCC is "yoked" with the left anterior SCC. Thus, the SCCs work as a pair and the central nervous system (CNS) is always comparing the inputs from the right and left paired SCCs.

From a practical point of view, instead of giving you tips about the vestibular nerve, I would rather discuss this topic by reviewing a clinical approach to a giddy/dizzy patient.

In a patient complaining of "chakkar," the clinical history is the most diagnostic tool, particularly as there are no specific diagnostic tests and pathological confirmation if rare. Giddiness, dizziness, or "chakkar" is a very nonspecific term and can mean very different etiologies to different patients **(Table 9.1)**.

TABLE 9.1: Symptoms and Work-up in a patient complaining of *chakkar*/giddiness/dizziness.

Symptoms	Work-up
Light-headedness: • ? presyncope • ? vague	 • Cardiovascular • Nil
Imbalance of gait	Vestibular
	Cerebellar
	Peripheral neuropathy*
Seizure: Gets "dizzy" and falls unconscious	EEG, CTS, or MRI
Vertigo	EVE
Psychogenic	Counseling

(CTS: computed tomography scan; EEG: electroencephalogram; EVE: extended vestibular examination; MRI: magnetic resonance imaging)

*I have seen many patients who are diabetic and who complain of dizziness. They have usually seen their family physician who diagnosed them as vertigo. Thus, the patient starts using the word vertigo when reciting their symptoms. In spite of antivertigo therapy, which they have taken for several months or even up to 1–2 years, they do not get relief. Examination of the extraocular muscle (EOM) does not reveal any nystagmus. In such a situation, I do the Romberg test and when they are swaying with their eyes closed, because of a sensory ataxia, I ask them, "is this your dizziness or vertigo?" Invariably, their answer is yes. Kindly note that in such cases, a sensory ataxia can be misinterpreted as dizziness, giddiness, or vertigo. Therefore, it is very important to ask the patient to describe their symptoms *without* using words like dizziness, giddiness, vertigo, or "chakkar". In this manner, you are very likely to establish whether the patient has "true" vertigo or other vague symptoms as described above.

Once you have established the true nature of vertigo, the key elements in history are precipitating factors, tempo and duration, accompanying features, and a list of medications that they are taking.

- *Precipitating factors*: If vertigo is precipitated from the supine to the sitting or standing-up position, the problem is very likely orthostatic hypotension, particularly if the patient has diabetes. If the patient complains of vertigo on lying down and turning to one side, it is benign paroxysmal positional vertigo (BPPV). Note that the lower ear is the abnormal ear and in the majority of cases, it is the posterior SCC which is at fault. If the precipitating factor is quick head movements associated with blurred vision, the likely etiology is acute or chronic bilateral vestibular hypofunction. Lastly, if straining at stools or lifting a heavy weight precipitates vertigo, it is very likely a perilymph fistula.
- *Duration of symptoms*: The duration of vertigo is a fairly good indicator of the etiology as shown in **Flowchart 9.1**.
- *Tempo of symptoms*: Symptoms of vestibular disease tend to change over time. It is not uncommon for chronic vestibular disorders to initially present with severe vertigo and then merge into a less well-defined symptoms of visual disorientation. Hence, a detailed description of the initial attack is often the best indicator of the etiology.
- *Accompanying symptoms*: Hearing loss, tinnitus, and aural fullness are reliable indicators of a peripheral disease. Acute vertigo with accompanying hearing loss is indicative of viral labyrinthitis or involvement of the internal auditory artery. In the earlier days, this situation would raise the possibility of syphilis, particularly in young males. Episodic tinnitus with hearing loss is very characteristic of MD. Lastly, distortion of sound and autonomic symptoms, pallor, sweating, nausea, and vomiting, favor an acute peripheral vestibular disease. On the other hand, if these symptoms are accompanied by loss of consciousness, hemiparesis, headaches, seizures, and cranial nerve palsies, the CNS is involved.
- *Medication*: In the elderly, particularly ask for prolonged use of "sleeping tablets." Benzodiazepines and antiseizure medications are known to produce symptoms of vertigo. Antihistamines and scopolamine are also incriminating medicines.

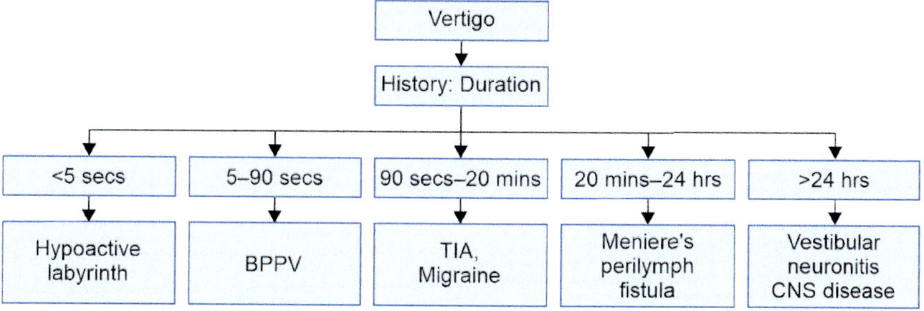

FLOWCHART 9.1: Etiologies of vertigo and their duration.

Note: The differentiating points between MD and vestibular neuronitis are already mentioned earlier.

(BPPV: benign paroxysmal positional vertigo; CNS: central nervous system; TIA: transient ischemic attack)

Clinical Examination

Clinical examination is divided into two parts, a standard neurological examination and an extended vestibular examination (EVE). The main purpose is to detect either vestibular imbalance or bilateral vestibular hypofunction. The most useful diagnostic sign is nystagmus.

Tips during examination of nystagmus: I have already covered this earlier in the chapter of Oculomotor Nerves, but some tips are worth reiterating.

- Nystagmus is dampened by convergence. Hence, keep your finger or torch at least 14 inches away.
- If the nystagmus is minute, shine a torch on the conjunctiva. The enhanced reflection makes small movements more visible.
- For torsional movements, do not concentrate on the iris/pupils. Look at the small conjunctival blood vessels. Their up/down movements will make torsional nystagmus more evident.
- Nystagmus in the primary position is dampened by fixation—the examiner's finger. Ask the patient to look at a totally blank wall and then ask him/her to look to the right or left.

The standard neurological examination will not only establish the presence of nystagmus but will also detect other accompanying signs which will help to differentiate between peripheral and central vertigo.

Nystagmus:

- Spontaneous nystagmus is detected either in the primary position of the eyes or during conjugate gaze—gaze-evoked nystagmus.
- Nystagmus in the primary position is practically pathognomonic of vestibular imbalance. The CNS interprets the imbalance as movement, inducing a VOR. Thus, the eyes move slowly in a direction opposite to that of the perceived movement. This is followed by the corrective saccade, i.e., nystagmus.
- The three key elements to study in nystagmus are (1) the amplitude, (2) the direction of the saccade, and (3) the effects of fixation **(Table 9.2)**.

TABLE 9.2: Characteristics of peripheral and central nystagmus.

Characteristics	Peripheral	Central
Type	Mixed H and/or V and/or T	Pure Only H, V, or T
Amplitude: In direction of fast phase	Increases	No increase
Direction: Change with gaze	Fixed	Changes
Fixation	Suppressed	Not suppressed

(H: horizontal; V: vertical; T: torsional)

- The characteristics of nystagmus of peripheral origin, lesions of the labyrinth or 8th nerve, are as follows:
  - *Type*: Mixed horizontal plus rotational/torsional nystagmus
  - *Amplitude*: It increases in the direction of the fast phase
  - *Direction*: It is fixed, i.e., it does not change with gaze. In an irritative lesion, the fast phase will be in the direction of the affected ear, whereas in a destructive lesion it will be toward the unaffected ear.
  - *Fixation*: The nystagmus is suppressed by fixation. Ask the patient to stare at a blank wall; nystagmus will be present. Then ask the patient to fix on your finger, the nystagmus stops. Suppression of nystagmus by fixation is at times called "fatiguable" nystagmus.
- The characteristics of nystagmus of central origin are as follows:
  - *Type*: Purely horizontal, vertical, or torsional.
  - *Amplitude*: It does not intensify in the direction of the fast phase.
  - *Direction*: This is changing, i.e., left beating nystagmus with left conjugate gaze and vice versa.
  - *Fixation*: There is no fixation suppression.

The common causes of peripheral vertigo are BPPV, MD, vestibular neuronitis, and ototoxic drugs. Common causes of central vertigo are migraine, lateral medullary infarct in the territory of posterior inferior cerebellar artery (PICA), cerebellar infarcts, and multiple sclerosis (MS). Note that CPA tumors like an acoustic neuroma rarely cause vertigo.

EVE: Specialized tests of vestibular function are beyond the scope of this book. I will only enumerate the tests and the information they give.

- *Hallpike-Dix test*: This is a maneuver which is specifically positive if a patient has BPPV. It is intended to stimulate the vertical SCC pair, i.e., the right anterior SCC and the left posterior SCC. In a normal person, nystagmus occurs during the change in position from sitting to supine and is very transient. In BPPV, the nystagmus starts at a latency of 4–10 seconds and lasts up to 30 seconds. This condition is very effectively managed by the simple canalith repositioning maneuver.
- *Head impulse test*: In a normal individual, the eyes do not move when the head is rotated from side to side. If you have vestibular imbalance, say the right ear is affected, the VOR is abnormal when the head is rotated to the right. You will see a corrective saccadic refixation when the head is brought from the right side to the midline position.
- *Dynamic visual acuity (V/A)*: The V/A is obtained with the head static and then oscillating at 2 Hz. Loss of three or more lines from the static V/A indicates vestibular dysfunction. This is a good test for bilateral vestibular hypofunctioning due to drug-induced ototoxicity or age.

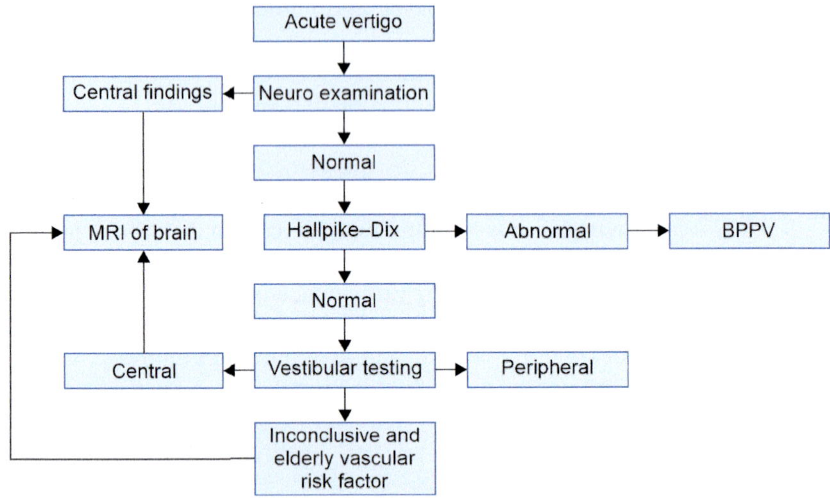

FLOWCHART 9.2: Algorithm of examination and investigation for acute vertigo.
(BPPV: benign paroxysmal positional vertigo; MRI: magnetic resonance imaging)

- *Head shaking test*: The head is pitched down 30° and oscillated horizontally. In an abnormal test, jerk nystagmus is elicited with the fast phase toward the stronger ear. This is a good test for vestibular imbalance.

In a case of acute vertigo, **Flowchart 9.2** is useful.

RECOMMENDED ARTICLES

1. Baguley D, McFerran D, Hall D. Tinnitus. Lancet. 2013;382:1600-7.
2. Brandt T, Dieterich M, Strupp M. Vertigo and Dizziness: Common Complaints, 3rd reprint. New Delhi: Springer; 2011.
3. Delaney KA. Bedside diagnosis of vertigo: the value of the history and neurological examination. Acad Emerg Med. 2003;10:1388-95.
4. Tusa RJ. Bedside assessment of the dizzy patient. Neurol Clin. 2005;23:655-73.

CHAPTER 10

Cranial Nerves 9 and 10: The Glossopharyngeal and Vagus Nerves

The glossopharyngeal nerve (GPN) is predominantly sensory, providing sensory afferents from the pharynx, tonsillar fossa, and soft palate. Its motor function (innervation of the stylopharyngeus—a pharyngeal elevator) is difficult to assess. The vagus nerve (VN) also provides sensations to the pharynx, larynx, ear canal, part of the pinna, and meninges of the posterior fossa. The sensory components of VN cannot be tested clinically as areas over the pinna overlap with other nerves, the meninges are inaccessible, and the epiglottis is difficult to test for taste. The motor component of the VN innervates the motor soft palate and the intrinsic muscles of the larynx.

For all practical purposes, the GPN and VN should be examined as a unit, the afferent arc of the gag and palatal reflex coming from the GPN and the efferent arc by the VN. The only component of the VN which is important in clinical practice and independent of the GPN is its parasympathetic innervation of the heart. The vagal tone is protective to the heart; it slows down the pulse and regulates the rhythm.

Gag reflex: Touching the posterior pharyngeal wall (GPN sensory) elicits a motor response (VN), involving tongue retraction with elevation and retraction of the pharyngeal wall.

Palate reflex: Touching the soft palate (GPN) elicits the motor response of elevation of the soft palate with the uvula in the midline (VN). Note that some individuals have a long and curved uvula. When the palate is elevated, it may give a false impression of deviation to the side opposite to the curve. In such cases, look at the spot where the uvula meets the soft palate.

Lesions involving the GPN and VN will be considered together except when they involve only one of them.

Supranuclear lesions: Unilateral lesions are not important as they produce no deficit because of bilateral supranuclear innervation. Bilateral lesions are usually associated with pseudobulbar palsy of any etiology—vascular or neurodegenerative. The gag reflex is markedly exaggerated. In small vessel disease (lacunar infarcts) or neurodegeneration [motor neuron disease (MND)], the earliest feature is that the patient gags or coughs repeatedly while having his meals, particularly liquids. When pseudobulbar palsy is suspected in the history, this must be asked for particularly from the caregiver. Pseudobulbar palsy is also a feature of primary lateral sclerosis—a variety of MND. The patient usually presents with spastic dysphonia and dysphagia. Most of the investigations, including magnetic resonance imaging (MRI), are normal. Although this variety of MND is suspected with the above symptoms, it is very difficult to prove electrophysiologically. I have had one patient in whom four electromyographies (EMGs) performed at an interval of 6–8 months failed to show chronic partial denervation in the limbs. It is only when the patient progressed and became anarthric, that the fifth EMG showed evidence of denervation in the tongue and lower limbs.

Unilateral paralysis of the GPN/VN is rarely in isolation and usually decided by the "anatomical company" they keep. The motor symptoms are usually that of a nasal twang and the soft palate is pulled to the normal side. The classical example is the plethora of findings with palatal palsy in the Wallenberg syndrome [anterior inferior cerebellar artery (AICA) infarct]. In the posterior fossa, these two nerves together with the spinal accessory nerve can get involved at the jugular foramen—Vernet syndrome—especially by glomus jugulare tumors. As these tumors tend to bleed in the middle ear, they give a bluish discoloration to the tympanic membrane, a clinical finding to suspect glomus jugulare tumors. Bilateral involvement produces weakness of the soft palate, pharynx, and larynx. The voice is hoarse and the cough is weak. I frequently use a good cough as an indicator of normal motor functions of the larynx and therefore of the VN. Dysphagia is also a prominent symptom, particularly for liquids.

An important point I would like to stress is bilateral VN involvement in Guillain-Barré syndrome (GBS). In early involvement, the voice is hoarse and the patient is only able to use short telegraphic sentences. On saying "aah", frothy salivary secretions are seen with weak palatal movements. The cough is weak, indicating motor laryngeal involvement. Another point, which is often not stressed, is that because of lack of parasympathetic vagal tone, there is sustained tachycardia. These are warning signs that the patient may require assisted ventilation. Hence, it is always prudent to monitor the pulse/heart rate in a patient with GBS. At times, tachycardia is so prominent that I have given beta blockers to slow down the heart rate and prevent arrhythmias. Lastly, the first indication that the patient is ready to be weaned off a ventilator is the spontaneous reduction in the tachycardia. These are useful points in the management of GBS in the intensive care unit.

Two disorders involving these cranial nerves deserve a mention here:

1. *Glossopharyngeal neuralgia (GPNg):* The important point about GPNg is that the pain is lancinating like in trigeminal neuralgia but occurs deep within the mouth and radiates to the ear and angle of the mandible. It is aggravated by swallowing and in each individual, the attacks are stereotypical.

2. *Recurrent laryngeal nerve (RLN)*: This branch of the VN has a long intrathoracic course, the left being longer than the right. This makes the left RLN more prone to injuries from various intrathoracic etiologies. Isolated RLN palsy produces a harsh dysphonia due to paralysis of all the intrinsic laryngeal muscles, except the cricothyroid which is supplied by the superior laryngeal nerve. Hence, any case of so-called idiopathic dysphonia needs imaging of the thorax, as the etiologies may be life-threatening like aneurysm of the thoracic aorta or metastasis from breast carcinoma.

With bilateral RLN palsy, there is severe approximation of the vocal cords producing inspiratory stridor and dyspnea on exertion, necessitating tracheostomy.

CHAPTER 11

Cranial Nerves 11 and 12: The Spinal Accessory and Hypoglossal Nerves

SPINAL ACCESSORY NERVE

During development, the motor neurons from the motor nucleus of the vagal nerve migrate to the anterior horn cells of C1–4 segments of the cervical cord. The spinal accessory nerve (SAN) arises from the ventrolateral part of the C1–4 segments, and they ascend as a common trunk and enter the cranial cavity through the foramen magnum to merge with the trunk of the accessory nerve. The SAN then exits through the jugular foramen, together with the glossopharyngeal nerve (GPN) and vagus nerve (VN), and descends in the neck to innervate the sternocleidomastoid (SCM) and the trapezius (TPZ) muscles. The innervation of the SCM is mainly from the C2 segment, the upper third of the TPZ from the accessory nerve, and the lower two thirds from the C3–4 segment. These anatomical facts have a bearing in the denervation of the TPZ muscle.

Lesions of the Spinal Accessory Nerve

From a practical point of view, supranuclear and intramedullary lesions almost never occur. If at all there is a C1–4 cervical cord injury, the involvement of the SAN is masked by the other signs of an upper cervical cord lesion.

Ipsilateral injury to the SAN is common due to penetrating injuries by bullets or knives in the neck. This is more in war zones and unlikely in peace times. It can also be injured by adenopathy, particularly matted glands in the posterior triangle of the neck and by neoplasms in the same location. Iatrogenic injury of the SAN is not uncommon during surgery in this area and in one retrospective series the most frequent injury involved lymph node biopsy. This is of relevance in India where lymph node biopsies are performed frequently for tuberculous lymphadenopathy. With paralysis of the SCM muscle, the patient is unable to move the face to the normal side but can do so to the affected side. Bilateral SCM weakness produces weakness of the flexion of the neck against resistance (pressure applied to the forehead or lower part of the chin).

Because of the pattern of innervation, the paresis due to SAN injury predominantly affects the upper fibers of the TPZ muscle (those parts not supplied by the C3–4 segments). Involvement of the upper fibers of the TPZ results in downward and lateral displacement of the scapula, atrophy of the superior one third of the muscle, and "winging" of the medial border of the scapula. When the patient is asked to stand with both upper limbs loosely at the sides, the affected side droops lower. This is evident by observing the fingertips which are at a lower level on the affected side. The displacement of the scapula may be better demonstrated by asking the patient to bring his upper limbs in front of him with the palms together. The fingertips on the affected side will protrude further. Besides the droop, there is winging of the scapula which will be discussed in detail in Chapter 12: The Motor System. Bilateral TPZ paresis results in neck extension weakness. The head tends to fall forward when the patient attempts to stand erect. The SAN can be involved intracranially but is almost never isolated and is diagnosed by the involvement of the neighboring 9th and 10th cranial nerves.

HYPOGLOSSAL NERVE

The main functions of the tongue are taste, speech, and food manipulation in the mouth. Taste is subserved by the chorda tympani branch of the facial nerve (anterior 2/3rd) and the GPN (posterior 1/3rd). The four intrinsic muscles of the tongue are primarily involved in changing the shape of the tongue while speaking. The most peculiar feature of these muscles is that they have no bony attachments—they arise and are inserted within the tongue. Food manipulation in the mouth is done by the extrinsic muscles, namely genioglossus, styloglossus (retrusion and elevation of the lateral margins), hyoglossus (retrusion and depression of the latera margins), and palatoglossus, which elevate the posterior part of the tongue, close the oropharynx, and initiate swallowing. From a practical point of view, the most important muscle supplied by the hypoglossal nerve is the genioglossus which protrudes the tongue. It can also poke the tongue into the inner part of the cheek, and thus the power of the genioglossus can be tested.

Unilateral paralysis hardly ever produces any functional disturbance except that the tongue deviates to the affected side on protrusion and is atrophic. Bilateral paresis occurs most commonly in pseudobulbar [upper motor neuron (UMN)] or bulbar [lower motor neuron (LMN)] palsy **(Fig. 11.1)**. The speech is initially indistinct (try talking while holding your tongue or willfully keeping it immobile). Later, particularly in bulbar palsy, the patient becomes anarthric. Additionally, in bulbar palsy, fibrillations of the tongue are seen. One should ask the patient to open his mouth without attempting to protrude the tongue to check for fibrillations. If he attempts to protrude the tongue, pseudo-fibrillations are seen even in normal individuals who are tense. Further, the flaccid paretic tongue may fall back when the patient is supine and give rise to snoring. Hence, recent onset of snoring

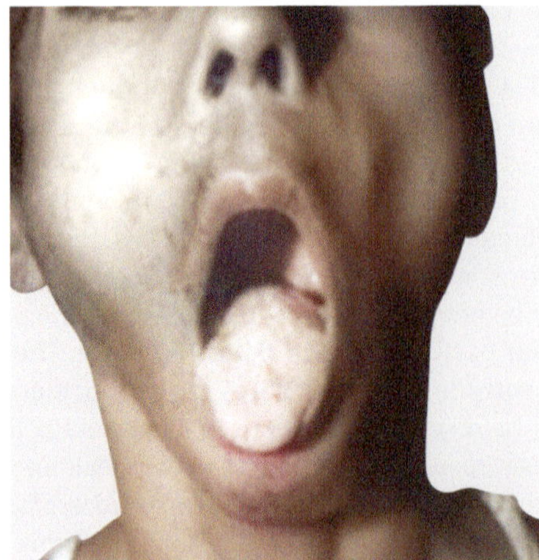

FIG. 11.1: Same patient as in Figure 8.2 showing an atrophic tongue.

in an elderly individual deserves attention and investigations. In the later stages of bulbar palsy, the tongue is atrophic and lies immobile in the base of the mouth.

RECOMMENDED ARTICLE

1. Kim DH, Cho Y-J, Tiel RL, Kline DG. Surgical outcomes of 111 spinal accessory nerve injuries. Neurosurgery. 2003;53:1106-13.

CHAPTER 12

Some Topics from the Motor System

The motor system is a hierarchal system. It consists of many long tracts within the central nervous system, but the main one that we have to examine is the corticospinal tract (CST) or more popularly known as the pyramidal tract. The upper motor neuron (UMN) component of the CST begins at the Betz cells in the cerebral cortex and innervates the motor nuclei of the cranial nerves (the corticobulbar tract) and the anterior horn cells (AHC) in the spinal cord (the corticospinal tract). The lower motor neuron (LMN) component begins at the AHC in the spinal cord. The other components are the anterior roots within the spinal canal, mixed roots, peripheral nerves, myoneural junction (MNJ), and the muscle—the motor component of the peripheral nervous system. The activity of the CST is modulated by the extrapyramidal system (EPS) with inputs originating from the basal ganglia, cerebellum, vestibulospinal, and rubrospinal systems for posture. The reticulospinal system maintains tone in the antigravity muscles through modulation of the "fusimotor" tone of the tiny gamma motor neurons.

At the level of the spinal cord, the CST ends on the motor unit of the cervical, thoracic, lumbar, and sacral AHC giving rise to a segmental level of involvement; for example, involvement at the C5 level of the cervical cord will give rise to LMN signs due to the involvement of the motor unit at that level and UMN signs below that level. Here, I would like to reiterate that besides the axons of the alpha motor neurons, the anterior roots also contain the axons from the small gamma motor neurons, which play an important role in maintaining muscle tone by innervating the intrafusal muscle fibers of the muscle spindle.

Traditionally, the motor system examination involves:

- Presence of absence of wasting
- Testing muscle tone:
  - Hypertonia—UMN lesion, spasticity, or rigidity
  - Hypotonia—LMN lesion
- The main symptoms of weakness

Dealing with the entire motor system is again beyond the scope of this book. I will only deal with a few selected topics which in my opinion have intrigued postgraduates and young neurologists (including me in the early stages of my career).

TOPIC 1: PATTERN OF INVOLVEMENT OF THE CORTICOSPINAL TRACT

Cortical Lesions

It is important to remember that lesions situated in the cerebral cortex hardly ever fail to involve the subcortical white matter. These two levels share a functional relationship, and consideration of a "pure" cortical lesion is artificial and hardly ever seen clinically. For this reason, predominantly cortical lesions will be expressed as "cortical." These lesions produce monoplegia.

- *Facial monoplegia*, i.e., only the lower face is predominantly involved.
- *Upper limb monoplegia*: As the hand area has a greater cortical representation, it is more paretic than the forearm, arm, or shoulder.
- *Lower limb monoplegia*: This involves the rostral part of the paracentral lobule. It produces a predominantly foot weakness resembling a "foot drop." However, the ankle tone is spastic, the ankle jerk is exaggerated, and the plantar response is extensor. This clinical scenario is not uncommon with parasagittal meningiomas. I have seen an elderly lady with this typical clinical picture who was seen by three orthopedic surgeons and advised surgery for a L4-5 disc lesion based on a lumbar magnetic resonance imaging (MRI). When I advised an MRI of the brain, the elder sister of the patient had a very skeptical look and expressed her feeling in no uncertain terms. Fortunately, they got the MRI done and the elder sister was very apologetic because it showed a parasagittal meningioma.

Apart from the above clinical scenario, spasticity in cortical lesions, particularly due to strokes, is less pronounced and rarely produces contractures. Such patients may have focal seizures with a "Jacksonian" march. If the postcentral gyrus is involved, various sensory phenomena may occur—parietal lobe syndromes.

Subcortical Lesions

Level of the Centrum Semiovale

As the fanned-out cortical fibers become more compact, the motor disturbances are wider. Therefore, at this level, there is more than a monoplegia but less than a hemiplegia, unless the lesion is very large and extends deeper to involve the internal capsule (IC). At this level, there is hemiparesis with a predominant faciobrachial involvement or lower limb > upper limb > face. Spasticity is more in a subcortical lesion and can produce contractures if proper physiotherapy is lacking.

Level of the Internal Capsule

When the posterior limb of the IC is involved, it usually results in a dense hemiplegia with a hemisensory defect. This may be associated with a homonymous hemianopia if the lesion extends more posteriorly and caudally to involve the optic tracts.

Acute lesions of the subcortical centrum semiovale (CSO) or IC initially produce a flaccid, areflexic hemiplegia. There is a conjugate deviation of the eyes away from the hemiparesis (looking to the side of the lesion), characteristic of a hemispheric lesion (see Fig. 6.6 on page 51).

Level of the Diencephalon

The diencephalon (Latin for between brain) lies between the cerebrum (telencephalon) and the midbrain. It has two major components: Thalamus and hypothalamus. Disorders of the hypothalamus do not produce any CST abnormalities and will not be considered here.

Lesions of the CST at the level of the diencephalon mainly involve the thalamus in ischemic or hemorrhagic strokes. The thalamus is strategically located at the rostral end of the brainstem and because of its complex anatomy and vascularization, it produces a variety of ischemic and hemorrhagic stroke syndromes. An understanding of the vascular anatomy and the regions that they supply is essential to understand the clinical findings in patients with thalamic infarcts of hemorrhages. Although all the lesions do not involve the CST, they will be considered here as thalamic strokes.

The vascular territories of the thalamus are divided into four major areas and shown in **Table 12.1**.

Lateral Thalamic Infarcts

Lateral thalamic infarcts in the territory of thalamogeniculate arteries can produce three common clinical syndromes:

1. *Pure sensory stroke*: The onset is with paresthesia or numbness on one side of the body. The sensory involvement is slight and involves a part of the hemibody, e.g., face plus upper limb (UL) or UL, trunk, and lower

TABLE 12.1: Vascular territories of the thalamus.

Arteries	Origin	Region supplied
Thalamogeniculate	6–10 tiny vessels from P2 segment of PCA	Ventrolateral
Polar	PComA	Anterolateral
Thalamo-subthalamic	P1 segment of PCA or common stem from BA (Percheron)	Medial
Posterior choroidal	P2 segment of PCA just distal to TG	Pulvinar and posterodorsal

(BA: basilar artery; PCA: posterior cerebral artery; PComA: posterior communicating artery; TG: thalamogeniculate artery)

limb (LL). Months later, a delayed painful syndrome occurs in the affected area. Although this stroke does not involve the CST, it has been included here for ease of understanding.

2. *Sensory-motor stroke*: The same sensory symptoms and signs described above are accompanied by ipsilateral paresis. This syndrome occurs with lateral extension of the infarct into the posterior limb of the IC adjacent to the ventrolateral nuclei of the thalamus.
3. *Large infarct of the lateral thalamus*: Large infarcts in this area produce the "thalamic syndrome"—pure sensory or sensorimotor strokes are associated with abnormal movement disorders, cerebellar hemiataxia, inability to stand and walk, and a delayed hemidystonia. Cognition and behavior are characteristically preserved in lateral thalamic infarcts.

Polar Artery Infarcts

The infarcts in this territory produce predominantly neuropsychological disturbances.

Paramedian Thalamic–Subthalamic Artery Infarcts

Unilateral infarcts in this territory produce a classic triad of symptoms—acute deterioration in the level of consciousness ranging from lethargy, difficulty in arousing, hypersomnolence, and even coma simulating a metabolic disorder. In addition, there is a vertical gaze palsy. This is characteristically seen as the "sunset eyes" of thalamic infarcts or hemorrhages in this area. The last component is neuropsychological abnormalities. These become evident as the patient becomes more alert after the acute phase. He/she may be disoriented and apathetic. Amnesia is prominent, and confabulations are common.

Patients who have a single artery of Percheron develop infarcts bilaterally in the paramedian thalamic-subthalamic area. In these patients, the neuropsychological abnormalities are more severe and long-lasting. Neuroimaging gives the classical "spectacle" infarcts.

Infarcts in the Territory of the Posterior Choroidal Artery

The characteristic findings are homonymous quadrantic or hemianopic defect due to the involvement of the posterior geniculate body. Impairment of ipsilateral pursuits may be present due to involvement of the pulvinar.

Thalamic Hemorrhages

Thalamic hemorrhages may be small (<2 cm) or large (>2 cm). Small thalamic hemorrhages behave exactly like thalamic infarcts. Large thalamic hemorrhage is one of the most common sites of hypertensive intracerebral hemorrhage (ICH). It usually presents with a rapidly progressive hemiparesis with a hemisensory loss. Because of compression of the supranuclear vertical gaze pathways in the rostral tectal region of the midbrain, vertical gaze palsy results. Clinically, this is manifest as tonic downward gaze deviation with convergence—the characteristic "sunset" eyes. In addition, the pupils are small, fixed, or sluggishly reacting to light. In contrast to thalamic infarcts, in thalamic hemorrhages, the motor deficits are more prominent.

Level of the Brainstem

One of the hallmarks in the localization of brainstem lesions is the "alternate" character of the involvement: Ipsilateral signs due to involvement of motor or sensory cranial nerve nuclei or other nuclear masses and contralateral long tracts (usually CST) signs. The ipsilateral signs will denote the level of the brainstem lesion—midbrain, pons, or medulla. There can be no doubt as to the side, level, and position (dorsal/ventral, medial/lateral) of the lesion when consideration is given to the cranial nerve nuclei and long tracts affected—pyramidal tracts, medial lemniscus, spinothalamic tracts, or a combination of two of them.

Among the long tracts, the motor tracts are descending whereas the sensory tracts are ascending. For the undergraduates, I compare these long tracts, particularly the CST, to railway tracks and the cranial nuclei or intraparenchymal fibers of the cranial nerves as railway stations. Lastly, as far as the motor system is concerned, I will essentially consider lesion of the CST/pyramidal tracts. These are mainly in the tegmentum (ventral aspects) of the brainstem. Therefore, pure tectal (dorsal) lesions, as a rule, do not produce any motor paralysis. Unfortunately, there are always exceptions to the rule with very large lesions.

Lesions of the Midbrain (Figs. 12.1A and B; Table 12.2)

The important structures in the midbrain are: (1) Crux cerebri containing the medial corticobulbar, corticospinal, and lateral corticobulbar tracts; (2) nuclei of the 3rd and 4th cranial nerves, together with the intraparenchymal 3rd nerve fibers, particularly those subserving the pupillary light reflex; (3) substantia nigra and red nucleus; and (4) the rostral part of the medial longitudinal fasciculus (MLF).

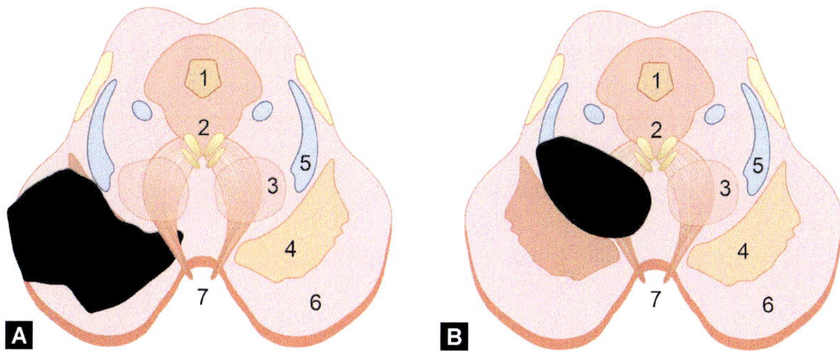

FIGS. 12.1A AND B: Midbrain syndromes. (A) Weber; (B) Benedikt.

Structures are: (1) Cerebral aqueduct, (2) oculomotor nucleus (note that the MLF is just anterolateral to it and the trochlear nucleus just caudal to it), (3) red nucleus, (4) substantia nigra, (5) medial lemniscus, (6) crux cerebri, and (7) oculomotor nerves in the interpeduncular region.

TABLE 12.2: Known stroke syndromes in the midbrain.

Midbrain structure	Syndrome	Signs
Crux cerebri	Weber	Ipsilateral 3rd nerve palsy, contralateral hemiplegia
Tegmentum (red nucleus)	Benedikt	Ipsilateral 3rd nerve palsy, contralateral hemiataxia

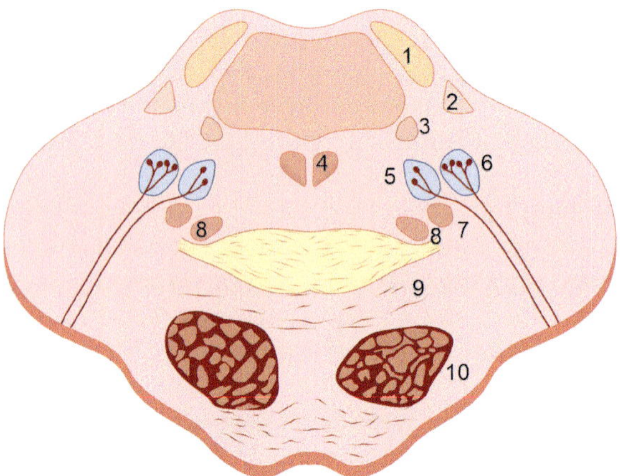

FIG. 12.2: Section through mid-pons, showing important structures at the level of the trigeminal nucleus.

Structures shown are: (1) Middle cerebellar peduncle, (2) lateral spinothalamic tract, (3) bulbothalamic tract, (4) MLF, (5) motor nucleus of trigeminal, (6) principal sensory nucleus, (7) rubrospinal tract, (8) superior olivary nucleus, (9) medial lemniscus, and (10) corticobulbar and corticospinal tracts.

Lesions of the Pons (Figs. 12.2 and 12.3; Table 12.3)

The important structures in the pons are: (1) Corticobulbar and corticospinal tracts, (2) abducens nucleus together with its intraparenchymal fibers producing either a lateral rectus (LR) or lateral conjugate gaze palsy, (3) facial nucleus and its intraparenchymal fibers with their peculiar orientation around the abducent nucleus producing a combination of ipsilateral LR and facial palsy. In addition, we have the 5th nerve nuclei in the tegmentum of the mid-pons as follows:

- *Principal sensory nucleus*: Involvement may produce anesthesia/ hypesthesia of the ipsilateral face.
- *Nucleus of the sensory tract*: Impaired pain/temperature over ipsilateral face.
- Motor nucleus, just medial to the principal sensory nucleus, produces difficulty in mastication and deviation of the jaw to the affected side on opening the mouth.

Thus, the nature of the involvement, motor or sensory, in the distribution of these cranial nerves (5th, 6th, 7th) will indicate the level of involvement of the CTS in the pons.

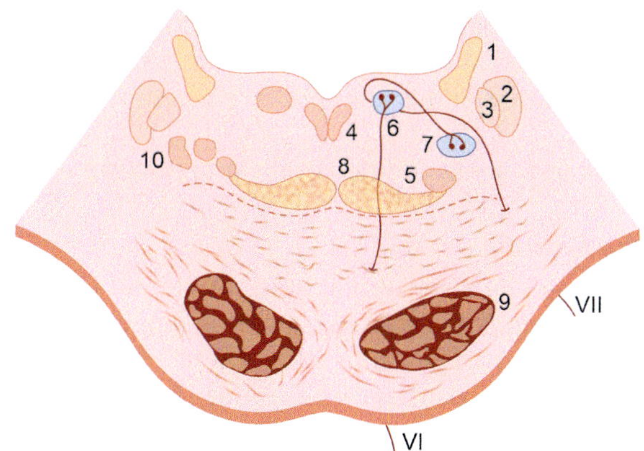

FIG. 12.3: Section through lower pons at the level of the abducens and facial nuclei.

Structures shown are: (1) Superior vestibular nucleus, (2) spinal tract of trigeminal, (3) spinal nucleus of trigeminal, (4) MLF, (5) superior olivary nucleus, (6) abducens nucleus, (7) facial nucleus and nerve (note the peculiar relationship to the abducens nucleus), (8) corpus trapezoideum and medial lemniscus, (9) corticobulbar and corticospinal tracts (note rostral to caudal as well as transverse fibers), (10) rubrospinal tract (shown only on the left for convenience), (VI) emerging abducens, and (VII) facial nerves.

TABLE 12.3: Known stroke syndromes in the pons.

Pons	Syndrome	Signs
Inferior, medial and more ventral tegmentum	Millard–Gubler	IL 6th nerve (intra-axial fibers) and face CL: Hemiplegia
Inferior, medial and more dorsal tegmentum	Foville	IL: LR or CG palsy and face CL hemiplegia*

Note: MGS and FS are more frequently observed with hemorrhages or in the early phases of brainstem gliomas. They are uncommon with vertebrobasilar ischemic strokes.

(CG: conjugate gaze; CL: contralateral; IL: ipsilateral; LR: lateral rectus)

*I have always been intrigued by the overlap between the Millard–Gubler syndrome (MGS) and Foville syndrome (FS). They share common physical findings, namely ipsilateral 6th nerve palsy or conjugate gaze palsy, ipsilateral facial nerve palsy, and contralateral hemiplegia. Therefore, distinction between FS and MGS is difficult. However, the more ventral location of the lesion in MGS catches the intra-axial part of the abducens nerve, whereas the more dorsal location of the FS involves the abducens nucleus and the adjacent parapontine reticular formation (PPRF). Thus, in my opinion, FS can present with either ipsilateral LR palsy (abducens nucleus involvement) or a conjugate lateral gaze palsy together with the other two features. If the 6th nerve nucleus is involved, then the conjugate gaze palsy is masked. As the intra-axial part of the abducens nerve is involved, MGS involves ipsilateral 6th and 7th nerves together with contralateral hemiplegia.

Another important "anatomical neighbor" of the CST in the tegmentum of the pons is the medial lemniscus, conveying proprioceptive sensations to the thalamus. Lesions at this level produce contralateral hemiplegia with contralateral proprioceptive loss. Such patients are severely handicapped, not only by weakness, but in addition by the proprioceptive loss.

Lesions of the Medulla

The size of the medulla is small and hence, small lesions can give rise to marked loss of function. A classic example is Wallenberg syndrome (lateral medullary infarct) due to a posterior inferior cerebellar artery (PICA) lesion. Important tracts and nuclei in the medulla which help in localizing the lesion are as follows:

- *Site of the decussation of the CST*: A tiny lesion involving the lateral part of the decussation produces a rare "cruciate hemiplegia"—ipsilateral upper limb (crossed fibers to the upper limbs) and contralateral lower limb (uncrossed fibers to the lower limb) **(Fig. 12.4)**. To be absolutely honest, in all my years of practice, I have not seen a single case of cruciate hemiplegia and it is only of anatomical/historical significance. A midline lesion of the pyramidal decussation will produce spastic weakness of all four limbs but spares the face, and the sensations are normal. This type of lesion may simulate a high cervical cord lesion, which is more commonly seen than the former, which is rare.

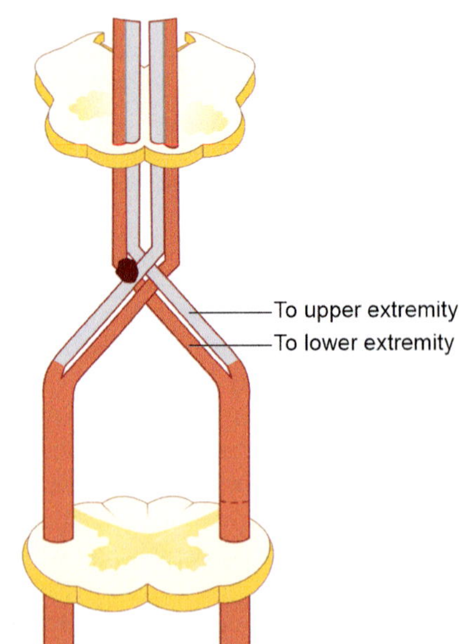

FIG. 12.4: Unilateral lesion (black dots) producing a cruciate hemiplegia.

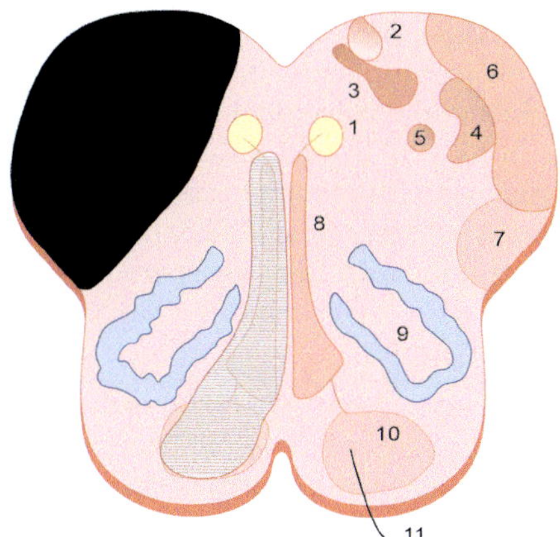

FIG. 12.5: Medullary infarcts. Shaded area is medial and black area is lateral (Wallenberg syndrome).

Structures involved are: (1) Hypoglossal nucleus, (2) medial vestibular nucleus, (3) vagus nucleus, (4) spinal tract of trigeminal, (5) spinal nucleus of trigeminal, (6) inferior cerebellar peduncle, (7) spinothalamic tract, (8) medial lemniscus, (9) inferior olivary nucleus, (10) corticospinal tract, and (11) emerging hypoglossal nerve.

- Medially placed lesions extending from the pyramidal tracts dorsally, to just anterior to the floor of the 4th ventricle (**Fig. 12.5**, gray area). Such lesions produce a contralateral hemiplegia (CST), contralateral hemi proprioceptive loss (medial lemniscus), and ipsilateral tongue involvement (hypoglossal nucleus or intraparenchymal fibers).
- *Lateral medullary lesion* (**Fig. 12.5**, black area): Although the lateral medullary syndrome does not involve the CST, it is the most common syndrome localizing to the lateral medulla and is therefore considered here. There are a plethora of symptoms and signs:
  - *Vertigo*: Medial vestibular nucleus involvement
  - *Ipsilateral palatal palsy*: Vagal nucleus
  - *Ipsilateral ataxia*: Involvement of the inferior cerebellar peduncle (restiform body)
  - *Ipsilateral facial hemianesthesia*: Spinal tract of the 5th nerve
  - *Contralateral hemianesthesia*: Involvement of the ascending spino-thalamic tract
  - In addition, some patients may have an ipsilateral Horner syndrome

It may be noted that many patients develop partial Wallenberg syndrome and it is rare to have all the components in one patient. If so, the prognosis for good recovery is guarded.

Pseudobulbar Palsy

Pseudobulbar palsy (PBP) is commonly secondary to multiple lacunar infarcts involving bilateral corticobulbar and corticospinal tracts. The classical form of PBP involves these tracts at the upper pontine level (above the decussation of the corticobulbar tracts to the face). This produces the classical signs of emotional lability and exaggerated facial as well as deep tendon reflexes. The patient also has swallowing problems with gagging, particularly with liquids. Rarely PBP is due to bilateral involvement of the CSTs below the level of the facial nucleus in the pons. PBP in such cases produces features in difficulty in swallowing and gagging with bilateral exaggerated deep tendon reflexes (DTR). However, there is no emotional lability or exaggerated facial reflexes as the corticobulbar pontine projections are spared.

Level of the Spinal Cord

From a practical point of view, the spinal cord is divided into 30 segments: 8 cervical, 12 thoracic, 5 lumbar, and 5 sacral. Each segment has a motor and sensory root which merge just before or at the intervertebral foramina. Taking the metaphor of the railway tracks and stations, the CST in the lateral white matter of the spinal cord are the tracks and each root on either side from the stations. Thus, there are 30 "railway stations" on either side, throughout the length of the "railway tracks."

A few principles must be understood when trying to localize lesions at the spinal cord level:

- Spinal cord lesions will have UMN signs below the level of the lesion and LMN signs at the level of the lesion, if the AHC or the anterior roots are involved.
- Paralysis of a group of muscles, which have the same radicular innervation, localizes the lesion to the AHC or anterior root, thereby localizing the level of the spinal cord involved.
- Cutaneous radicular zones in the limbs are longitudinally located, whereas over the trunk they are circular in orientation. During embryonic development, radicular zones of the limb buds are at right angles to the trunk. As the limb buds grow, these zones become displaced longitudinally along the limbs **(Fig. 12.6)**.

Thus, mapping of the sensory impairment in the limb is more difficult than over the trunk. To ease your task, refer to the examination of the

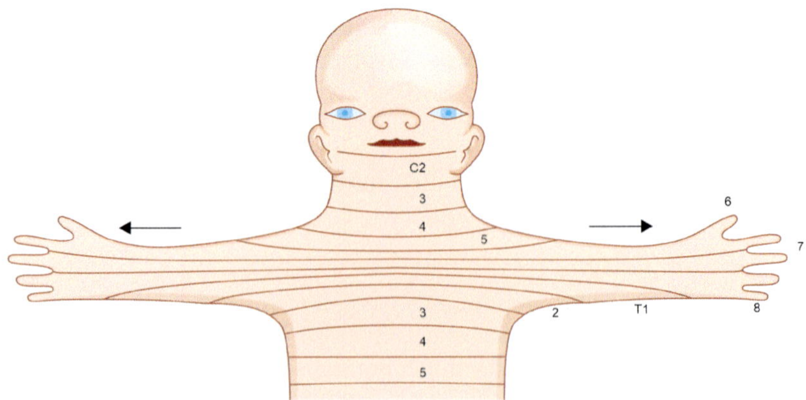

FIG. 12.6: Longitudinal displacement of dermatomes in the formation of the upper limb.

radicular lesions in the sensory system. Establishing a sensory level over the trunk is easy and gives an accurate spinal cord level. For example, a sensory level at the umbilicus signifies a T10 spinal cord lesion and a sensory level at the nipples in males signifies a T4 level.

- Each radicular sensory field overlaps with the adjoining radicular field. The overlap is such that anesthesia can occur only when two or more roots are involved, whereas hypesthesia may occur when only one root is involved.
- Muscles affected in damage at various levels in the spinal cord are shown in **Table 12.4**.
- As a rule, localizing value of the DTR is good, but those of the superficial reflexes is not.
- The alignment of the spinal cord segments and that of the vertebral segments are shown in **Table 12.5** and **Figure 12.7**. At birth, the spinal

TABLE 12.4: Movement/muscles affected at various levels of the spinal cord.

Levels of spinal cord	Movement/Muscles affected
Cervical: Upper	• Neck/Head movements • Elevation of the shoulders
Cervical: Middle	• Diaphragmatic breathing • Movement of upper arm/forearm
Cervical: Lower	Hand and finger movements
Thoracic	• Intercostal muscles • Abdominal muscles
Lumbar: Upper	• Flexion at the hip • Adduction of the thighs
Lumbar: Lower	• Other movements of thighs • Movements of the leg
Sacral	• Movement of the foot and toes • Contraction of the sphincters and perianal muscles

TABLE 12.5: Correlation between spinal cord and vertebral level.

Sensory level: Spinal cord	Vertebral level
Cervical e.g., C8	Minus 1 C7
Thoracic: T1 to T6 e.g., T6	Minus 2 T4
Thoracic: T7 to T12 e.g., T12	Minus 3 T9
Lumbar 1, 2	T10
Lumbar 3, 4	T11
Lumbar 5	T12
Sacral/Coccygeal	L1

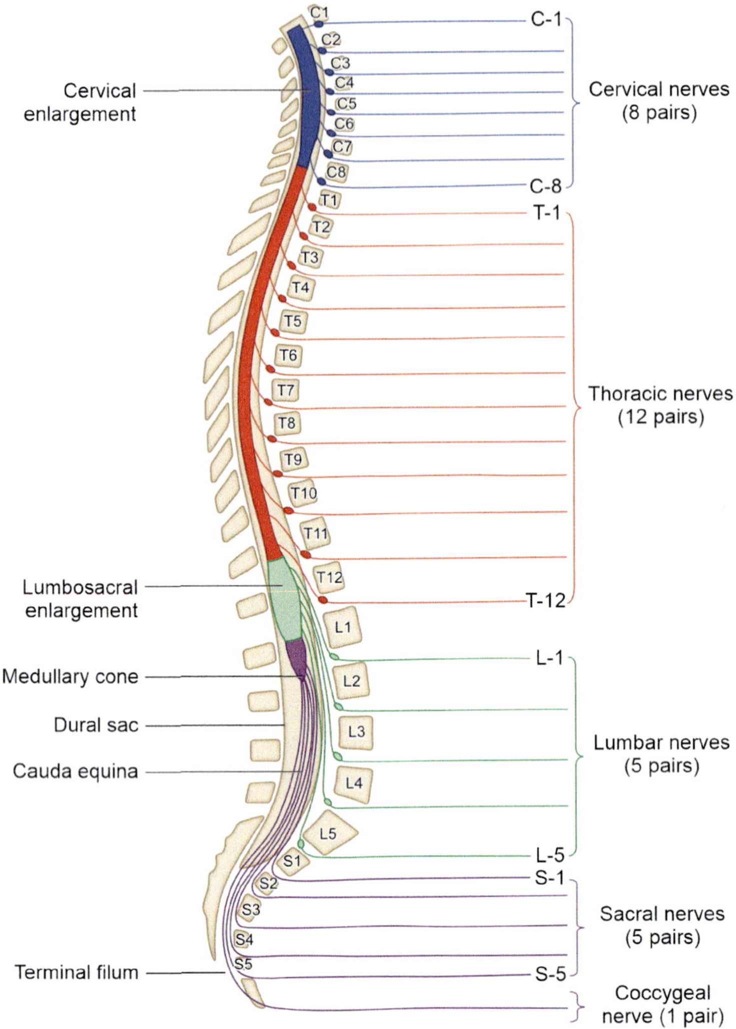

FIG. 12.7: Correlation between the spinal cord and vertebral levels.

cord ends at the level of L3. Subsequently, the growth of the vertebral column outstrips the growth of the spinal cord. Therefore, in adults, the spinal cord so-called ascends within the spinal canal and ends at the mid-level of L1 vertebra. Hence, there is no spinal cord in the lumbar canal beyond L1. Yet, time and again, I have seen patients with a spastic paraparesis coming with a lumbar spine X-ray or MRIs, ordered by either internists or orthopedic surgeons.

Thus, a combination of motor and sensory signs gives an accurate localization of the CTS in a spinal cord lesion.

TOPIC 2: PERIPHERAL MOTOR SYSTEM: LOWER MOTOR NEURON

This part of the motor system consists of the following:

- *Anterior horn cell (AHC) and anterior roots*: For all practical purposes, the disorders encountered are essentially of the AHCs. The main disorders to consider are: (1) Acquired: Motor neuron disease (MND), (2) Inherited: Spinal muscular atrophy (SMA), and (3) Infections: Poliomyelitis and other polioclastic disorders like EV-70 disease.
- *Roots and plexopathies.*
- *Peripheral neuropathies*: These are commonly acquired and uncommonly inherited. Pathologically, they may be axonal or demyelinating (usually treatable). They are commonly motor/sensory, but some may be purely or predominantly motor at onset **(Box 12.1)**.
- *Myoneural junction (MNJ)*: The most common disorder is myasthenia gravis, but you may rarely see autoimmune Lambert–Eaton myasthenic syndrome or botulinum toxicity from eating contaminated tinned food.
- *Muscle disorders*: Clinically, the most commonly occurring disorders are the dystrophies, inflammatory myopathies, and drug-induced myopathies. These disorders can be classified as:
    - *Inherited*: Dystrophies, congenital myopathies, mitochondrial myopathies, and channelopathies (rare)
    - *Inflammatory*: Dermatomyositis, polymyositis, inclusion body myositis
    - *Endocrine*: Hypo-/hyperthyroidism, pituitary dysfunction, hypo-/hyperparathyroidism, osteomalacia, primary hyperaldosteronism
    - *Drug induced*: Statins, fibrates, corticosteroids, colchicine, antimalarial drugs, zidovudine, alcohol

BOX 12.1 Peripheral neuropathies with predominantly motor symptoms at onset.

Motor symptoms on presentation/predominantly motor:

- GBS, CIDP, AMAN
- Lead intoxication
- Acute porphyria
- Hereditary M-S neuropathy (CMT)
- MMN*, MADSAM
- Diphtheria, neuroborreliosis
- *Toxic*: Dapsone, amiodarone, vincristine, nitrofurantoin
- *Endocrine*: Thyrotoxicosis, hyperparathyroidism

*MMN is the only disorder in this list, which is purely motor.

(AMAN: acute motor axonal neuropathy; CIDP: chronic inflammatory demyelinating polyneuropathy; CMT: Charcot–Marie–Tooth; GBS: Guillain–Barré syndrome; MADSAM: multifocal acquired demyelinating sensory and motor neuropathy; MMN: multifocal motor neuropathy; M-S: motor-sensory)

TABLE 12.6: Important muscles of the upper limbs (ULs).

Area	Muscle	Root value	Nerve
Shoulder			
Abduction	First 20° supraspinatus *Rest*: Deltoid	C5 C5, 6	Suprascapular Circumflex
Adduction	Pectoralis major	C6, 7, 8, T1	Lateral and medial pectoral
External rotation	Infraspinatus	C5, 6	Suprascapular
Elbow			
Flexion Forearm midprone	Biceps Brachioradialis	C5, 6 C5, 6	Musculocutaneous Radial
Extension	Triceps	C7, 8	Radial
Forearm			
Pronation Supination	Pronator teres Supinator	C6, 7 C5, 6	Median Radial
Wrist			
Extension Flexion	Extensor carpi radialis longus Extensor carpi ulnaris Flexor carpi radialis Flexor carpi ulnaris	C7, 8 C7, 8 C6, 7, 8 C7, 8	Radial Radial Median Ulnar
Fingers			
Long flexors	Proximal interphalangeal joint (PIPJ) flexor digitorum sublimis Distal interphalangeal joint (DIPJ) flexor digitorum profundus (Digits 1 and 2) (Digits 3 and 4)	C7, 8, T1 C8 C8	Median Median Ulnar
Long extensors	Extensor digitorum	C7, 8	Radial

The important muscles to be examined in the upper and lower limbs, together with their root value and nerve innervation, are shown in **Tables 12.6 and 12.7**.

Muscles of the Hand

- *Muscles of the thumb*: Thenar–flexor pollicis brevis (FPB), abductor pollicis brevis (APB), and opponens pollicis (OP). Root value C8, T1, median nerve:
  - Adductor pollicis brevis. Root value C8, T1, ulnar nerve
  - Extensor pollicis brevis. Root value C7, 8, radial nerve

- *Muscles of the little finger*: Hypothenar–flexor, abductor, opponens digiti minimi. Root value C8, T1, ulnar nerve
- *Dorsal and palmar interosseous*: Root value C8, T1, ulnar nerve
  [*Note*: Early wasting is detected in the 1st dorsal interosseous (DIO)]
- *Lumbricals*:
  - Digits 1 and 2: Root value C8, T1, median nerve
  - Digits 3 and 4: Root value C8, T1, ulnar nerve

  Note: Isolated wasting of the thenar muscles is due to median nerve palsy.

  Isolated wasting of the 1st DIO is due to ulnar nerve palsy.

  Wasting of both is more likely to be due to C8, T1 root lesions unless there is trauma at the elbow involving both the median and the ulnar nerves.

TABLE 12.7: Important muscles of the lower limbs.

Area	Muscle	Root value	Nerve
Hip			
Flexion	Ilio-psoas	L 2, 3	Femoral
Abduction	Gluteus medius/minimus	L4, 5, S1	Superior gluteal
Adduction	Adductors–brevis, longus, magnus	L2, 3, 4	Obturator
Extension	Gluteus maximus	L5, S1, 2	Inferior gluteal
Knee			
Extension	Quadriceps	L 2, 3, 4	Femoral
Flexion	Hamstrings	L5, S1	Sciatic
Ankle			
Dorsiflexion	Tibialis anterior	L4, 5	Sciatic
Plantarflexion	Gastrocnemius	S1, 2	Sciatic
Inversion	Tibialis posterior	L4, 5	Sciatic
Eversion	Peroneus longus/brevis	L5, S1	Sciatic
Toes			
Flexion	Flexor hallucis longus Flexor digitorum longus	S1, 2 S2	Sciatic Sciatic
Extension	Extensor hallucis longus Extensor digitorum longus Extensor digitorum Brevis	L5, S1 L5, S1 S1	Sciatic Sciatic Sciatic
Small muscles of the foot*		S1, 2	Sciatic

*The action of the small muscles of the foot is to produce flexion and simultaneous adduction of the toes.

A few facts and clarification about MND would be in order here. The most common variety of MND is amyotrophic lateral sclerosis (ALS) which has some degree of overlap with progressive bulbar palsy (PBP). The hallmark of ALS is progressive weakness in the presence of UMN and LMN signs. In 35% the disease begins in the upper limbs, in 30% in the lower limbs, and in 30% of the cases there is a bulbar onset. For the clinical diagnosis, it should affect more than one anatomical region: Cervical, thoracic, lumbar, or bulbar (tongue). In corticobulbar onset, dysarthria invariably precedes dysphagia. If dysphagia occurs simultaneously with dysarthria, the disease is more aggressive. During the course of ALS, at least 80% will develop bulbar involvement. Bilateral wasting of the lateral tongue is the rule in the late stages of the disease and aids in electrophysiological confirmation.

PBP: It is an unsatisfactory terminology and fails to capture the full spectrum of clinical heterogeneity of ALS. As mentioned above, 30% of cases of ALS have a bulbar onset. Middle-aged men who develop a bulbar onset of the disease have a more aggressive disease. In limb-onset ALS, the prognosis is better irrespective of the fact whether it began in the upper or lower limbs.

Progressive muscular atrophy (PMA): Only a small percentage of patients will show only LMN signs. PMA is the term reserved for such cases. It is rare, and most of them will develop UMN signs later in the disease; thus, it is more appropriate to call them "LMN-predominant MND." Often, the degree of wasting is out of proportion to the extent of weakness.

Primary lateral sclerosis (PLS): MND with only UMN signs is termed PLS. Again, such cases are rare. Clinically, they present with ascending quadriparesis with a spastic dysarthric speech in the majority. Primary progressive multiple sclerosis (PPMS) is a close differential diagnosis and should be ruled out by MRI. When the patient presents with only UMN signs, there is difficulty in establishing the diagnosis electrophysiologically (see case of primary lateral sclerosis in Chapter 10, page 72). Thus, it would be appropriate to call them "UMN predominant MND."

Motor neuron disease is a cause of a "dropped head." The other common etiologies are myasthenia gravis and dermatomyositis. Such patients complain of severe pain in the nape of the neck as the extensors have to work extra to maintain the upright position of the head. In some of these cases, particularly MG, I have advised them to wear a soft cervical collar in order to support the chin. This gets rid of the pain in the nape of the neck.

SPECIAL TOPICS IN THE MOTOR SYSTEM

- Subtle hemiparesis
- Winging of the scapula
- Examination of the thenar muscles of the hand
- Differentiating myopathies from neurogenic disorders

Subtle Hemiparesis

I have found several maneuvers useful in detecting subtle hemiparesis.

You all know about the pronator drift and I will not dwell on it further. Hachinski and Norris described the following manoeuvres, which I have found useful. Ask the patient to keep his upper limbs outstretched in front of him with the hand extended at the wrist and the fingers adducted. Then ask the patient to close his eyes. After a while, the little finger and thumb will abduct on the weaker side. Another manoeuvre which I have used frequently because it is very rapid and easy to perform is as follows: Ask the patient to elevate both upper limbs in front of him, with the palms facing downward and his eyes closed. Tap his upper limbs gently at the wrist, alternatively. On the weaker side, the downward excursion of the limb will be more. The neurologist involved in the care of strokes may find these maneuvers useful.

Lastly, in cases of reversible ischemic neurological deficit (RIND) who come to you for a follow-up later, there is hardly any neurological deficit. In such cases, I "titrate" the deep tendon reflexes (DTRs), particularly the knee jerks, to lateralize to the abnormal size. This is further described in Chapter 14: Understanding Tone and the Deep Tendon Reflexes.

Winging of the Scapula

Normally, the medial/vertebral border of the scapula is flat against the posterior thoracic wall. Two muscles are responsible for this: the trapezius muscle (TZM) and the serratus anterior muscle (SAM). With weakness of either of these two, the entire vertebral border of the scapula protrudes backward like a wing—winging of the scapula.

Trapezius winging: An important anatomic fact to remember here is that the upper one-third of the TZM is innervated by the accessory nerve and C2 root and the lower two-thirds by the C3 and C4 roots. Because of this pattern of innervation, the TZM is predominantly involved either in its upper one-third or lower two-third segments. In the upper one-third involvement, when the upper limb is relaxed, the scapula is displaced downward and laterally due to overaction of the lower two-third of the muscle. The upper limb on the affected side droops downward, which can be noted by observing the fingertips when the arms are relaxed at the sides of the body. Secondly, on asking the patient to bring his arms forward, with the palms together, the fingertips on the affected side project further forward.

Involvement of the lower two-thirds of the TZM produced more obvious winging, but the scapula is displaced upward and laterally due to the unopposed action of the upper one-third of the muscle.

Trapezius winging is accentuated when the arm is abducted laterally against resistance. Another method is to ask the patient to adopt the "starting block" pose of a swimmer during races—the upper body is flexed at the waist and arms are raised to the side and extended. This again accentuates the winging. But note that the winging practically disappears when the patient is asked to elevate the upper limb forward and press against a wall.

Serratus anterior winging: The SAM is innervated by the long thoracic nerve (root values C5 to 8). The SAM is known as the "boxer's muscle" as it keeps the scapula flat against the posterior thoracic wall when the boxer jabs his opponent—upper arm flexed forward forcefully. In contrast to the trapezius winging, the SAM winging becomes more accentuated when the upper limb is flexed forward and pressed against the wall.

In facioscapulohumeral muscular dystrophy (FSHMD), both the trapezius and SAM are weak. Hence, the winging is very prominent. Because of weakness of the shoulder girdle muscles, both the shoulders droop downward and forward, displacing the lateral end of the clavicle downward. The patient has practically "horizontal clavicles," a sign that I use to suspect FSHMD as the patient sits in front of me.

ACTION OF THE MUSCLES OF THE THUMB

It is easy to demonstrate flexion/extension and abduction/adduction of the fingers. But I have observed that when an examiner asks a candidate to demonstrate the action of the various thumb muscles, the candidate often gets confused and makes mistakes. Certain anatomical facts make this task very simple:

- There are four muscles which move the thumb—three of which form the thenar eminence and the adductor pollicis brevis. The thenar muscles are: flexor pollicis brevis (FPB), abductor pollicis brevis (APB), and opponens pollicis (OP).
  - *FPB*: It is the most medial muscle and has two heads—the superficial head supplied by the median nerve (T1) and the deep head supplied by the deep palmar branch of the ulnar nerve (C8-T1).
  - *APB*: This is the most superficial muscle and therefore early wasting is easily identified in carpal tunnel syndrome. It is supplied by the median nerve (T1).
  - *OP*: It lies deep to the APB. The opponens produce flexion, adduction, and medial rotation of the thumb. This action is very important for fine movements of the hand, for writing, or for pinching.
  - *The adductor pollicis has two heads*: The oblique and transverse. Its nerve supply is from the deep branch of the ulnar nerve (C8-T1).

The action of all these muscles is at the metacarpophalangeal (MP) joint. The most important fact to remember is the orientation of the thumb vis-à-vis the fingers and palm. Unlike the simian hand, the human thumb is oriented at 90° to the plane of action of the fingers. Then it is easy to depict the action of the various muscles which move the thumb.

- Flexion and extension of the fingers are perpendicular to the plane of the palm. Hence, FPB flexes the thumb in the plane of the palm. Extension is in the opposite direction and is done by extensor pollicis brevis (radial nerve, C6, 7, 8) in conjunction with the long extensors from the forearm.
- Abduction and adduction of the fingers is in the plane of the palm. Therefore, abduction and adduction of the thumb will be perpendicular to the plane of the palm. These actions are performed by the APB and the adductor pollicis, respectively. Abduction is away from the radial border of the palm and adduction is toward the base of the index finger.
- The action of the OP occurs when you touch the tip of the thumb to the MP joint of the little finger.

DIFFERENTIATING MYOPATHY FROM NEUROGENIC DISORDERS AT THE ANTERIOR HORN CELL LEVEL (SPINAL MUSCULAR ATROPHY)

Although localization of the lesion with motor and sensory deficits is relatively easy, it is difficult to differentiate between pure motor disorders like myopathy and SMA. **Table 12.8** shows some of the features that help to differentiate myopathies from such neurogenic lesions. Please remember that these are mere guidelines and there are many exceptions to the rule. Secondly, no single feature distinguishes one from the other (except for perhaps prominent pseudohypertrophy) and the sum of several features helps to distinguish one from the other.

TABLE 12.8: Clinical features of myopathy versus neurogenic lesion.

Features	Myopathy	Neurogenic lesion
Weakness at onset	Symmetrical	Asymmetrical
Pattern of weakness	Usually proximal	Distal +/– Proximal
Wasting and weakness	Weakness > Wasting	Wasting > Weakness
Pseudohypertrophy	+++	(+)
Fasciculations	(+)	+++
DTR in weak muscles	Lost late	Lost early
Gait	Toe walking + Waddling	Flat feet + Waddling
EDB	Usually preserved	Usually wasted
Tremors	Absent	Usually seen

[DTR: deep tendon reflexes; EDB: extensor digitorum brevis; (+): rare; +++: common; +/-: with/without]

EXCEPTIONS TO THE RULE

Weakness at onset: In distal myopathies as the name suggests, the weakness begins distally.

Weakness at onset: This may be asymmetrical in FSHMD.

Wasting: Inclusion body myositis shows prominent wasting, usually in the forearm muscles.

Fasciculations: These are occasionally seen in thyrotoxic myopathies.

In a study done in the Department of Neurology, Grant Medical College (GMC), and Sir JJ Group of Hospitals in 1969, the authors found that muscle percussion and 1 mg of neostigmine together with 0.6 mg of atropine given intramuscularly is useful in differentiating myopathies from neurogenic disorders.

Muscle percussion: The deltoid, quadriceps, or gastrocnemius muscles were sharply tapped with the triangular end of a percussion hammer and the response noted. A focal muscular contraction was seen in all the patients with neurogenic disorders but in very few patients with myopathies.

Neostigmine injection: Neostigmine-induced fasciculations were either exaggerated or unmasked in over 77% patients with a neurogenic disorder and in none of the cases with myopathy.

As the authors mention, neither of these two clinical tests are specific for differentiation but taken together with the other features mentioned in **Table 12.8**, are further helpful in differentiating myopathies from neurogenic disorders at the AHC level.

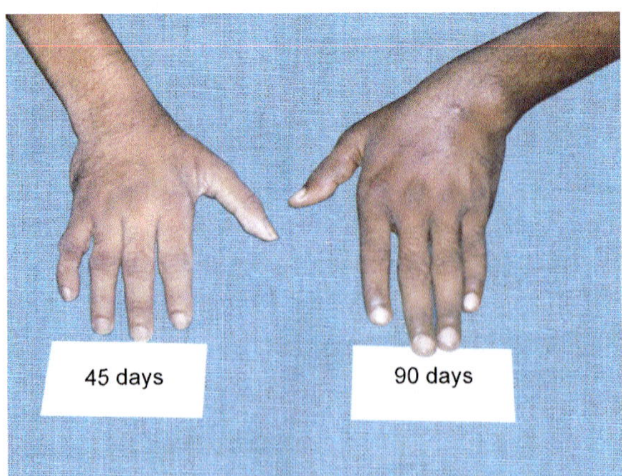

FIG. 12.8: Significant wasting in a patient with AMAN (left) compared to a patient with AIDP (right).

At this point, I would like to also mention my observation in differentiating axonal and demyelinating neuropathies. This observation is particularly relevant in differentiating demyelinating acute inflammatory demyelinating polyneuropathy (AIDP) (with a relatively good prognosis) from acute motor axonal neuropathy (AMAN). Early wasting, most obvious in the first dorsal interosseous, is a feature of axonal involvement, in contrast to hardly any wasting in demyelinating neuropathies **(Fig. 12.8)**.

Also note that multifocal motor neuropathy (MMN) and MND are pure motor disorders and therefore close differential diagnosis. In MMN, it being a demyelinating disorder, the weakness is out of proportion to the wasting whereas in MND, the reverse is true.

RECOMMENDED ARTICLES

1. Barth A, Bogousslavsky J, Caplan LR. Thalamic infarcts and haemorrhages. In: Bogousslavsky J, Caplan LR (Eds). Stroke Syndromes. New York: Cambridge University Press; 1995. pp. 276-83.
2. Hachinski V, Norris JW. Diagnosis of Stroke, Chapter 6. In Eds V. Hachinski and JW Norris, The Acute Stroke, FA Davis Company, Philadelphia, USA, 1985. pp. 79-101.
3. Patel AN, Swami RK. Muscle percussion and neostigmine test in the clinical evaluation of neuromuscular disorders. NEJM. 1969;281:523-6.
4. Silverman IE, Liu GT, Volpe NJ, Galetta SL. The crossed paralysis. The original brainstem syndromes of Millard-Gubler, Foville, Weber and Raymond-Cestan. Arch Neurol. 1995;52(6):635-8.
5. Talbot K, Turner MR. Amyotropic lateral sclerosis. In: Hilton-Jones D, Turner MR, Kennard C (Eds). Oxford Textbook of Neuromuscular Disorders. New Delhi: Oxford University Press; 2014. pp. 25-37.

CHAPTER 13

Some Topics from the Sensory System

The sensory system helps us stay in touch with the environment. Sensations are basically divided into: (1) special senses: smell, vision, taste, hearing, and vestibular function, which have already been covered with their respective cranial nerves, and (2) general somatic sensory modalities.

GENERAL SOMATIC SENSORY MODALITIES

General somatic sensory modalities are as follows:

- *Exteroceptive*: Information about the environment. Besides the special senses, this also involves somatosensory function of pain, temperature, and crude touch.
- *Interoceptive*: Information about internal environment. This is mainly a function of the autonomic nervous system and will not be covered here.
- *Proprioceptive*: Information about orientation of the body and limbs in space. It has a "conscious" component—the posterior columns subserving position and vibration sense and fine touch. These are conveyed by large myelinated fibers. The "unconscious" component is the spinocerebellar system, which subserves gait and posture.

Spinothalamic Sensations

The sensations of pain, temperature, and crude touch are conveyed by small myelinated fibers to the central nervous system (CNS) via the spinothalamic tract (STT) and the nucleus and tract of the trigeminal nerve **(Fig. 13.1)**. They terminate in the ventroposterolateral (VPL) and the ventroposteromedial (VPM) nuclei of the thalamus, respectively, which then projects to the sensory cortex. Itching and tickling sensations also go along these same tracts.

Proprioceptive Sensations

Position/vibration sense and fine touch are conveyed to the CNS by the posterior columns and medial lemniscus for the limbs and body and the

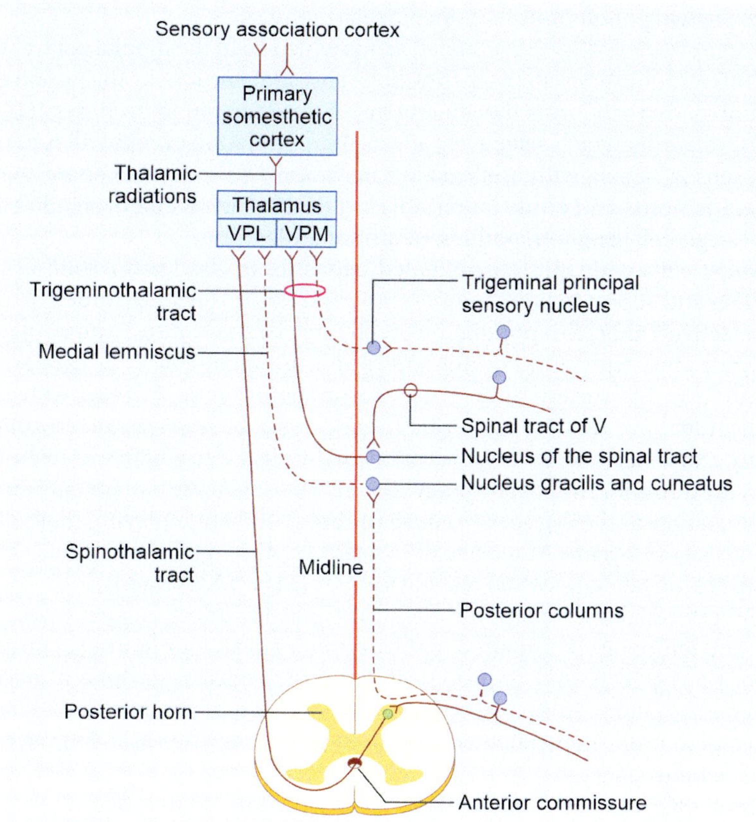

FIG. 13.1: Primary sensory tracts from the limb and face. Bold lines indicate pain/temperature and broken lines indicate proprioception.
(VPL: ventroposterolateral; VPM: ventroposteromedial)

principal sensory nucleus of the trigeminal nerve for the head and face **(Fig. 13.1)**.

These tracts terminate in the VPM and VPM nuclei of the thalamus, respectively, and are then projected to the post-Rolandic gyrus of the sensory cortex.

A few relevant anatomical facts must be mentioned here about the dorsal root ganglion (DRG). The DRGs lie on the posterior root at the intervertebral foramina just lateral to the point where the posterior roots pierce the dura. The DRG has unipolar cells; that is, a single axon leaves the cell body and then bifurcates into a peripheral and central component. This has implications in the "dying back" phenomenon of degeneration where there is a simultaneous central and peripheral component of degeneration moving toward the cell body of the DRG.

There are two populations of unipolar cells in the DRG:

1. Large cells with large myelinated axons which lie in the medial zone of the DRG and subserve vibration/position sense and fine touch. The peripheral limb of this cell forms the afferent arc of the deep tendon reflexes (DTR). Any disorder which selectively affects this population of cells will produce a sensory ataxia with areflexia but no motor weakness and spares pain, temperature, and crude touch. This "pattern" of involvement is indicative of large-cell ganglionopathies/neuronopathies.
2. Small cells with thinly myelinated axons lie in the lateral zone of the DRG and subserve pain, temperature, and crude touch. Disorders which selectively affect this population of cells are extremely rare. Paraneoplastic syndromes with anti-Hu antibodies due to small-cell lung carcinoma produce this variety of sensory neuronopathy. Rare families with this disorder have also been described and sporadic cases are even rarer. In all my years, I have seen only one case with this disorder, which was included in my thesis for DM in neurology. This 16-year-old male patient developed ulceration of the big toes because of shoe bites while playing football at the age of 12 years. At the age of 16 years, he developed ulcerations of the tips of the left hand while playing a guitar **(Figs. 13.2A and B)**.

On examination, he had the classical clinical features of such cases: (1) Pain and temperature impaired in the periphery of all four limbs, (2) normal motor power, DTR, and proprioception, and (3) normal peripheral nerves (PN) on palpation. These features can only localize to the small cells of the DRG and in India, they help to differentiate such rare cases from leprosy and diabetic neuropathy.

The DRG also has a highly vascular supporting stroma. Because of the vascularity, it is the weakest point of the nerve-cerebrospinal fluid (CSF) barrier and is prone to toxic, metabolic, and autoimmune disorders.

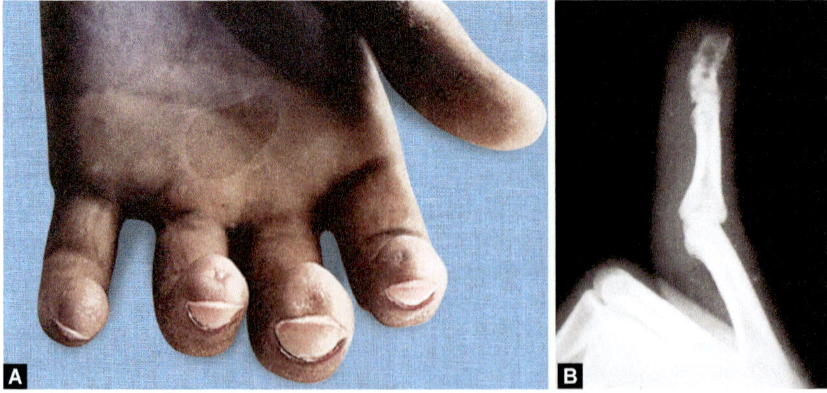

FIGS. 13.2A AND B: (A) Photograph of ulcers on the tips of the fingers; (B) X-ray of the right middle finger showing destruction of the terminal phalanx.

The general somatosensory modalities are divided into the following:

- *Primary modalities*: Pain/temperature sense, light touch and position, and vibration sense
- *Secondary/cortical modalities*: Two-point discrimination (2PD), stereognosis, graphesthesia, and tactile location

These modalities are usually affected due to parietal lobe disorders and apart from 2PD, they are beyond the scope of this book.

Pain and Thermal Sensations

These are carried by the STT. The nociceptive and thermoreceptors are the free or branched nerve endings in the skin. These sensations are carried by thinly myelinated Aδ and unmyelinated C fibers to the DRG. From the DRG, they enter the posterior gray horn, though some fibers may ascend one or two segments before entering the posterior horn. Here they synapse with the second-order neurons. The axon of these neurons crosses in the anterior commissure and forms the anterior and lateral STT (see **Fig. 13.1**). Because of this crossing, the sacral fibers are most lateral and the cervical fibers are most medial. Thus, with an expanding intraspinal tumor, the cervical, thoracic, and lumbar fibers are compressed first, with sparing of the laterally placed sacral fibers—the "sacral sparing" suggestive of an intramedullary lesion. The ascending STT maintains a lateral position in the medulla and pons, where they are frequently involved in a lateral medullary infarct.

Pain and thermal sensations from the head and face enter the pons via the Gasserian ganglion, descend in the spinal tract of the trigeminal nerve, and synapse in the adjacent nucleus of the spinal tract. They then ascend as the quintothalamic tract or trigeminothalamic tract (TTT). In the midbrain, the STT and the TTT converge and terminate in the VPL and the VPM nuclei of the thalamus, respectively.

Clinical Examination of Pain and Temperature

- To test pain, use any instrument sharp enough to produce pain but not sharp enough to draw blood. This is important as after the acquired immune deficiency syndrome (AIDS) epidemic, disposable instruments have been made available. This is really a waste of resources. I have used the sharp end of a toothpick or sharpened lead pencil to test for pain in human immunodeficiency virus (HIV) positive individuals. In HIV negative individuals, you can use the same instrument provided you do not draw blood.
- In an apprehensive patient (often encountered) or a child, an examination for pain should be done with their eyes closed.
- Always proceed from an area of low sensitivity to one of high sensitivity. This way you get a prompt response. Avoid giving the stimulus too rapidly or too close. This only serves to confuse the patient and make your work more difficult.

- These precautions are particularly useful in testing for dermatomal abnormalities. In the upper limbs (ULs), compare C5, 6 dermatomes (over the deltoid and lateral aspects of the arm) against the T1 dermatome (medial aspect of the arm). The difference, if any, will be very obvious. Similarly, in the lower limbs (LLs), compare L1, 2, 3 (front of the thigh) against S2, 3 (back of the thigh). Dermatomes also have a degree of overlap. Hence, a clear-cut border is not established, if one tests the dermatomes in sequence, i.e., C5–C6. When there is hypesthesia in the ophthalmic division of the trigeminal nerve, go beyond the intermeatal line (the line joining the right external auditory meatus to the left) on the scalp. The area behind this line is served by the C2 dermatome or occipital nerves and the contrast in pain will be obvious (low-sensitivity to high-sensitivity area). Watch the facial expressions. Some patients wince on reaching the sensitive area. Secondly, if a patient has functional numbness of the face, he or she mistakes the forehead and scalp as two different entities. The numbness may end at the border of the forehead with the scalp. Unfortunately, this is invalid in male patients with male pattern baldness. Fortunately, such patients are rarely functional.
- Temperature is tested by hot and cold tubes. In our department at JJ Hospital, Dr Wadia had made special stainless-steel tubes for this testing, with a plastic sleeve for the hot tube **(Fig. 13.3)**. Thermal modalities were tested by putting the tips of these tubes over the trunk and limbs.

From a practical viewpoint, thermal sense is equally affected as pain; hence rarely does it become necessary to test both. I would strongly recommend testing thermal sense when you suspect syringomyelia. The area of thermal loss far exceeds the impaired pain area and is easily detected.

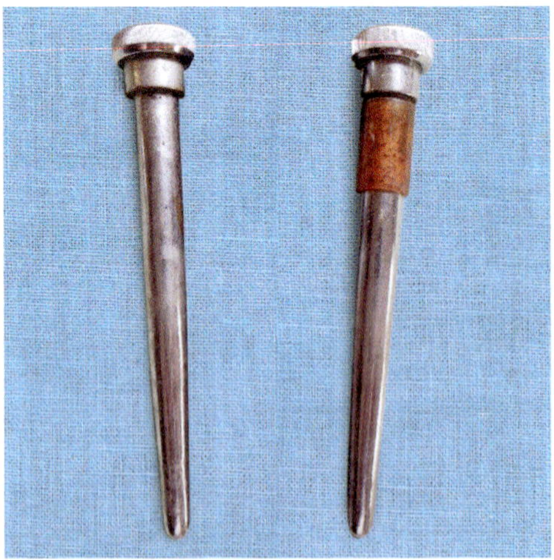

FIG. 13.3: Photograph of hot and cold tubes.

Case vignette

BMP male, 30 years. At the age of 27 years, he sustained a painless injury of the left index finger. Sepsis occurred and the finger was amputated. Following amputation, movement of the left wrist diminished and the wrist was swollen. He also complained of heaviness over the left UL and left side of the face. On examination, he had sensory hypesthesia in the left UL but a definite loss of thermal sensation from the second cervical segment to the third thoracic segment **(Figs. 13.4A and B)**.

Tactile Sensations

Many receptors are involved for tactile sensations. Therefore, this modality is conveyed by large and small myelinated fibers to the DRG. Fine discriminative touch is conveyed by the large myelinated fibers which are the peripheral arm of the large neurons in the DRG and ascend in the posterior columns whereas crude touch is conveyed by the STT. 2PD is a function of fine touch and thus the posterior columns.

Because of the duality of the pathways the general tactile modalities are lost late in spinal cord lesions, when other sensory clinical findings are very obvious. In contrast to that, light touch is lost early in peripheral neuropathies because of the range of receptors and myelinated fibers.

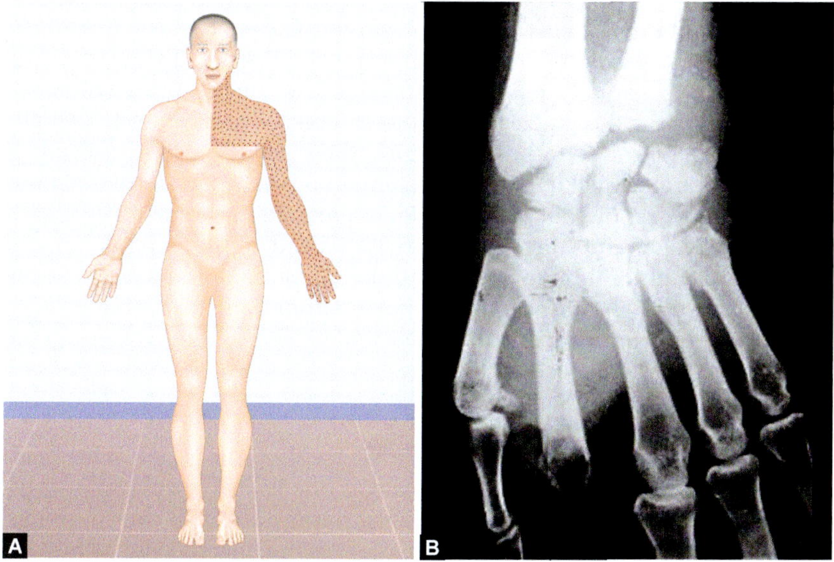

FIGS. 13.4A AND B: (A) Sensory charting showing a wider loss of thermal sensation; (B) X-ray of the left wrist: Disorganization of the wrist joint and note amputation of the left index finger.

Clinical Examination

- Light touch is tested by a wisp of cotton wool, a fine painting brush, or a piece of tissue paper. The most physiological fine touch is with the fingertips. Our first experiences of fine touch occur from the loving caresses of our mothers. I always use the tip of my index finger for fine touch.
- More detailed quantitative evaluation is not necessary in day-to-day practice but reserved for specialized clinics in diabetes and leprosy.

Two-point Discrimination

I personally believe that 2PD is a neglected modality of examination. I have found it particularly useful in patients with predominantly motor cervical radiculomyelopathy. The differential diagnosis in such cases lies between cervical spondylosis (a manageable condition) and motor neuron disease (an untreatable disorder). Test 2PD carefully in both little fingers. If the patient makes mistakes, you have a response which favors cervical spondylotic radiculomyelopathy. There is great joy when neurophysiological studies subsequently confirm your clinical diagnosis, and you earn the eternal gratitude of your patient.

Proprioceptive Sensations

Proprioceptive sensations involve position and vibration sense. The primary receptors are the muscle spindles with other receptors in the muscles, tendon, and joints, particularly the Pacinian corpuscles. Impulses from these receptors are conveyed by the largest myelinated fibers Ia to the DRG and ascend in the ipsilateral gracilis and cuneatus fasciculi (posterior columns). They terminate in the gracilis and cuneatus nuclei in the lower medulla. The axons of the second-order neurons then decussate and ascend as the contralateral medial lemniscus and end in the VPL nucleus of thalamus (see **Fig. 13.1**). All the fibers below T8 are grouped in the medially placed gracilis fasciculus and fibers rostral to T8 ascend on the laterally placed cuneus fasciculus. This is in contrast to the orientation of the fibers in the anterolateral STT. Proprioceptive impulses from the head and face go through the principal trigeminal nucleus and reach the VPM nucleus of the thalamus via the TTT.

Clinical Testing: Position Sense

- Position test is done by movement of the big toe at the metatarso-phalangeal (MTP) joint in the LLs and at the distal interphalangeal (IP) joints of the fingers in the ULs. A healthy young individual can appreciate a movement of 2–3° in the big toe and <1° in the fingers. With advancing age, this threshold increases.
- The fingers and toes should be grasped from the medial and lateral parts. Avoid pressure on the pulp of the fingers and toes.

- Quick movements of the joints are easily detected in comparison to very slow ones.
- *Romberg test*: This is a dynamic way of testing proprioception in the LLs and my preferred method of testing. To begin with, the patient should be able to stand with his feet together. In a patient with gross cerebellar ataxia with proprioceptive loss (Friedreich ataxia), this test cannot be performed. Some apprehensive patients may totter a lot when asked to close their eyes. In such cases, all I do is place the tips of my index finger on either shoulder. This is sufficient to assure the patient that I am around but not sufficient to steady them if proprioception is affected. With early affection of proprioception, the patient is able to maintain his posture with a lot of effort when the eyes are closed. This results in minute contractions of the tendons of the long flexors/extensors of the feet—the so-called dancing tendon sign.

Clinical Testing: Vibration Sense (VS)

- Strike a 128-Hz tuning fork and place it on a bony prominence. To establish a level, one can proceed proximally by going along bony points: Medial malleolus, tibial tuberosity, anterior superior iliac spine (ASIS), posterior spinous processes of the vertebrae, the ribs, wrist, elbow, and clavicle. From a practical point of view, after testing VS at the ASIS, jump directly to the lower rib cage.
- Please instruct the patient to appreciate the vibration and place the tuning fork over the forehead or sternum to know what normal vibration is. If not instructed properly, the patient may say that he feels something touching him.
- It is my experience that locally made aluminum tuning forks hardly vibrate. Buying a good-quality tuning fork is a once in a lifetime investment. I am still using my Weiss 128-Hz tuning fork, which I bought in Dunedin, New Zealand, in 1976. Lastly, avoid making a sound while striking the tuning fork.
- A normal young individual can feel the vibrations in the lower and upper limbs until it stops. VS particularly diminishes with age, and it is not unusual for an elderly patient to report absence of VS at the ankle. One can time the duration of the vibration, if one wants to be more accurate. This is maybe a useful method to document in patients of peripheral neuropathy, to judge improvement or deterioration on follow-up. A difference of >3–5 seconds between the two sides on successive examinations is considered abnormal.

Interoceptive (Visceral) Sensations

These are a function of the autonomic nervous system and are beyond the scope of this book.

Secondary or Cortical Sensations

The parietal lobe cortex is important in discriminating the finer grades of sensations such as the intensity of the sensation and the similarities and differences in the impulses which help in differentiating the form, weight, and texture of the object. This requires not only simple perception of the impulses, but also interpreting them with previously acquired concepts, e.g., differences in the "feel" of plastic material from a metallic one or the differences in the texture of cotton and silk. Thus, abnormalities of cortical sensory modalities are seen in lesions of the parietal lobes. They will be only enumerated here:

- *Stereognosis*: It is recognition and identification of the form and nature of an object by touch. Initially, the size and shape in two dimensions and the form in three dimensions are established. Then the object is identified from our previous experiences and concepts. Astereognosis can be diagnosed only if the primary sensory modalities (PSM) are normal.
- *Graphesthesia*: It is identifying letters and numbers written on the skin by a blunt object—like the tip of the examiner's index fingers.
- *2PD*: It is considered both as a delicate tactile modality and a more complex modality requiring parietal lobe interpretation. It has already been discussed earlier.
- *Sensory inattention*: It is inability to perceive two simultaneously applied stimuli on either side. One can use fine touch or pain. It is best to apply a light painful stimulus on one side then the other and judge the patient's response. If he correctly responds, "right and left," then the simultaneous impulses should be tested. On the abnormal side, the stimulus may be dull or absent, when applied simultaneously.
- *Spatial orientation*: Touch the patient on one side and ask him to point with his opposite index finger where he was touched. In the hand, this localization should be very precise.
- *Atopognosia*: This is a defect of body schema. The patient is unable to identify body parts. In the extreme form, the patient has been known to complain that somebody's upper limb (UL) has been left in their bed. A more restrictive disorder is the finger agnosia of the Gerstmann syndrome. The other features of this syndrome are right-left dissociation, acalculia, and agraphia. The features of this syndrome have been explained in a unique way. The acquisition of these various features begins in our childhood. We first learn to differentiate between right and left by using our dominant hand more. Calculations begin by counting the fingers of one and then the other hand. Later, with greater dexterity of the dominant hand, we start to write. If there is finger agnosia, all the other three features are lost. I feel this was a rather unique way to remember the features of Gerstmann syndrome.
- *Anosognosia*: It is the denial of the existence of a disease process; for example, the patient denies that he has hemiplegia. This is usually seen with the lesions of the nondominant parietal lobe.

PATTERNS OF PRIMARY SENSORY LOSS

- The PSM are involved in disorders of the PN, spinal roots, and sensory pathways in the spinal cord, brainstem, thalamus, and the cerebral hemispheres up to the level of the posterior limb of the internal capsule (IC).
- If the sensory pathways are in close anatomic proximity, then all modalities are affected—pain/thermal, fine touch, and proprioception. This happens in disorders of the PN, spinal roots, thalamus, and posterior limb of the IC.
- If the sensory pathways are not in close anatomic proximity, then one modality may be affected and the other spared, i.e., dissociated sensory loss. This occurs in disorders of the spinal cord and brainstem.
- Sensory and motor functions are interdependent and severe motor dysfunction can occur due to pure sensory impairment or due to involvement of the neighboring motor fibers/tracts. A patient with severe sensory ataxia has significant motor dysfunction, although on formal testing, the motor system is normal. In a spinal cord compression, the patient has paraplegia with a sensory level because of the close anatomical proximity of the motor and sensory pathways.

  These anatomical facts result in various patterns of primary sensory modality loss, depending on the level of the lesion, be it in the PN, spinal roots, spinal cord, brainstem, thalamus, or IC.
- In involvement of the peripheral part of the sensory system (PNs and spinal roots), the loss of the PSM occurs with lower motor neuron (LMN) signs. At all the other sites, besides the sensory loss, there will be upper motor neuron (UMN) signs. An exception to this rule is subacute combined degeneration (B12 myeloneuropathy) in which sensory loss is associated with both UMN and LMN signs.

Disorders of the Peripheral Nerves: Distal Symmetrical Sensory Loss

- The most common pattern is a distal symmetrical sensory loss of all the PSM. However, fine touch and vibration senses are affected first and the area of loss of fine touch is always more than that of pain.
- Uncommonly, the PNs may be pure sensory or predominantly sensory in their clinical presentation. In the purely sensory group, some may affect predominantly large myelinated fibers or the DRG producing a sensory ataxia and some may affect predominantly the small myelinated fibers producing a painful or painless neuropathy. Involvement of the small unmyelinated fibers produces significant autonomic symptoms and signs. The various etiologies of these characteristic neuropathies are shown in **Boxes 13.1 to 13.4**.
- The bulk of the PNs are axonopathies in which weakness with wasting is a prominent feature. Some PNs are predominantly demyelinating where the weakness is more than the wasting. A classic example is the

BOX 13.1 Neuropathies producing a sensory ataxia.

- Paraneoplastic anti-Hu syndrome (neuronopathy)
- Sjögren syndrome
- Idiopathic sensory neuropathy
- *Chemotherapy*: Cisplatin, thalidomide, vincristine, and doxorubicin
- HIV-related sensory neuropathy
- Lymphoma
- *Hereditary*: HSN/HSAN and Friedreich ataxia
- Megavitaminosis B6*
- SMON*

*Rarely or never seen nowadays.

(HIV: human immunodeficiency virus; HSAN: hereditary sensory autonomic neuropathy; HSN: hereditary sensory neuropathy; SMON: subacute myelo-optic neuronopathy)

BOX 13.2 Painful small fiber neuropathies.

- *Diabetes mellitus*: Burning feet syndrome and amyotrophy
- *Vasculitic neuropathy*: Can also be a MM
- Sjögren syndrome, sarcoidosis, and borreliosis (Lyme disease)
- Acute intermittent porphyria
- *Drug induced*: Isoniazid, arsenic, thallium, and antiretroviral
- HIV-related distal symmetrical neuropathy
- Alcohol/Nutritional
- *Inherited*: Amyloidosis, Fabry disease, and HSAN
- *Chemotherapy*: Bortezomib and thalidomide
- Cryptogenic sensory/sensorimotor neuropathy*

*Diagnosis made after excluding other etiologies.

(HIV: human immunodeficiency viruses; HSAN: hereditary sensory autonomic neuropathy; MM: mononeuropathy multiplex)

BOX 13.3 Painless neuropathies.

- Leprosy usually mononeuropathy or mononeuropathy multiplex
- *Diabetes mellitus*: Diabetic foot
- *Toxic*: Lead, usually mononeuropathy in upper limbs (ULs)
- *Familial/sporadic small-cell ganglionopathies*: Rare

BOX 13.4 Neuropathies with significant autonomic involvement.

- *Acute/subacute*: GBS, vincristine-induced, porphyria, and pandysautonomia (a rare variant of GBS)
- *Chronic*: Diabetes mellitus, Sjögren syndrome, HIV-related autonomic neuropathy, Toxic: arsenic, mercury, acrylamide, Inherited: amyloidosis, Fabry disease and HSAN, and paraneoplastic

(GBS: Guillain–Barré syndrome; HIV: human immunodeficiency viruses; HSAN: hereditary sensory autonomic neuropathy)

difference between Guillain-Barré syndrome (GBS) and acute motor axonal neuropathy (AMAN) (see Fig. 12.8 in Chapter 12, on page 96). Demyelinating neuropathies are potentially treatable with immune-modulatory therapies.

- There is an overlap between large fiber neuropathies producing a sensory ataxia and involvement of the large unipolar cells in the DRG (ganglionopathies or neuronopathies). The clinical features in favor of DRG involvement are severe sensory ataxia, minimal or no involvement of pain and temperature, and most importantly early absence of the DTRs in the presence of *normal* motor function.
- Mononeuropathies or mononeuropathy multiplex (MM) produces a unilateral or asymmetric loss of all PSM. Area of the sensory loss will correspond to the area of supply of that particular nerve. As already mentioned, the area of fine touch will be larger than the area for pain. Maps of areas of sensory loss for each specific nerve are available in many textbooks of neurology and even on the internet.

From a clinical viewpoint, the important nerves in the ULs are as follows:
Circumflex nerve: It supplies a coin-shaped area around the insertion of the deltoid. It is important to examine this area carefully in a suspected case of brachial neuritis.

The lateral (C5,6,7) and medial (C8, T1) cutaneous nerves of the forearm.

The *radial nerve* (C5–T1) has sensory areas above and below the elbow. The *median nerve* (C5–T1) and *ulnar nerve* (C8–T1) have areas below the elbow. From a practical point of view, in order to test the area of sensory loss of these three nerves, concentrate on the hand **(Figs. 13.5 to 13.7)**. The radial sensory loss is in the web on the dorsal aspect of the hand, between the

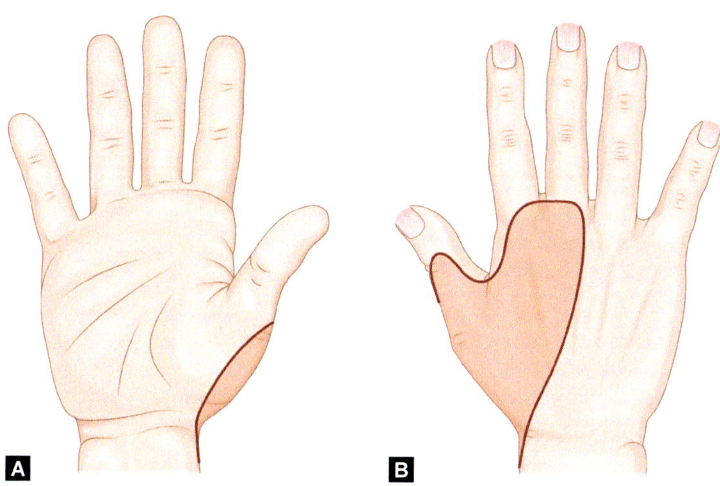

FIGS. 13.5A AND B: (A) Radial nerve palsy. (B) Area of sensory loss.

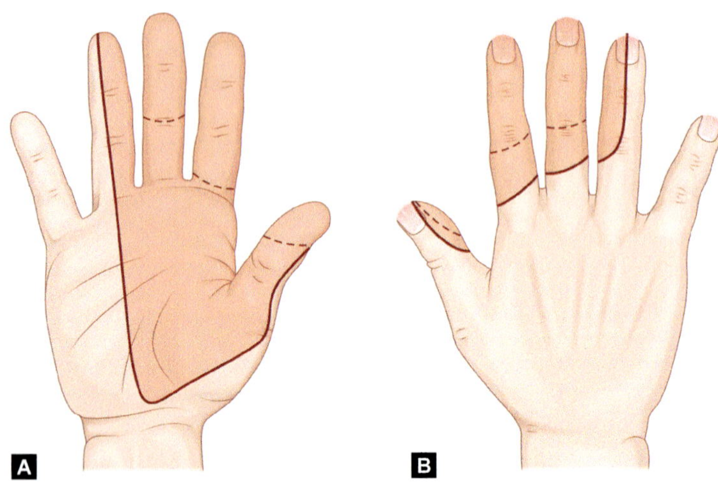

FIGS. 13.6A AND B: Median nerve palsy area of sensory loss.

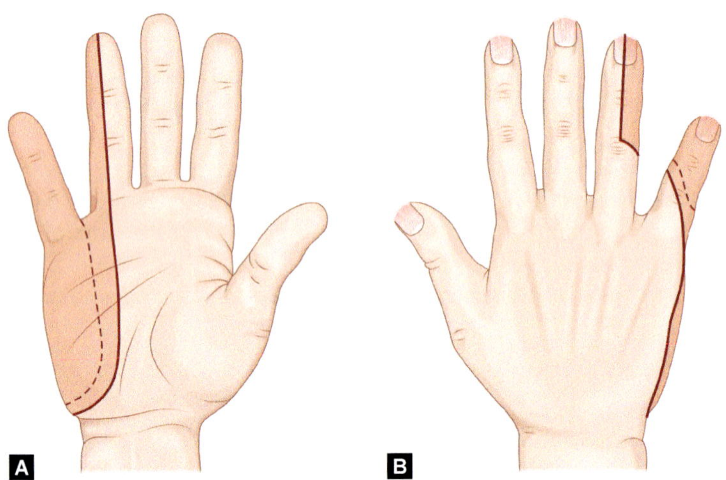

FIGS. 13.7A AND B: (A) Ulnar nerve palsy; (B) Area of sensory loss.

middle finger and the thumb. Note that there is a thin sliver on the palmar surface of hand as well. The common site of involvement is compression or trauma of the nerve in the radial groove of the humerus and there is an associated wrist drop.

The sensory loss of the median nerve is essentially on the palmar surface of the hand involving the thumb and the lateral two and a half fingers (lateral half of the ring finger). Note that it may involve the dorsal surface of these fingers distal to the proximal IP joint. Clinically, the most common etiology is the carpal tunnel syndrome, in which there will be early wasting of the abductor pollicis brevis (APB).

The ulnar nerve sensory loss involves both the palmar and dorsal areas of the medial part of the hand, involving the medial one-and-a-half fingers (the little finger plus the medial side of the ring finger). The most common site of involvement is in the ulnar groove of the humerus at the elbow—the tardy ulnar nerve palsy.

From a clinical viewpoint, the important nerves in the LLs are as follows:

- *Lateral cutaneous nerve of the thigh*: This nerve is entrapped in the tensor fascia lata on the lateral aspect of the thigh, producing meralgia paresthetica. There may be a large oval area of hypesthesia on the lateral aspect of the thigh.
- *Femoral nerve*: The most common etiology of this nerve's involvement is diabetic amyotrophy (unilateral) or diabetic proximal motor neuropathy (bilateral). Besides the severe pain and sensory loss over the anterior aspect of the thigh, there is weakness of the quadriceps and a sluggish to absent knee jerk in the former. Diabetic amyotrophy is a self-limiting illness and resolves within weeks or months with adequate control of diabetes. At times, with very strict dietary and diabetic control, the patient may complain of severe pain without sensory loss, along the anterior aspect of the thighs. This entity, known as diabetic cachectic neuropathy, is associated with severe weight loss. A more relaxed control of diet and diabetes resolves the issue. The femoral nerve can rarely get entrapped between the head of the fetus and pelvic floor in a patient with cephalopelvic disproportion and prolonged labor. Fortunately, because of the increase in the frequency of lower segment cesarean section (LSCS), this entity is rarely seen.
- *Lateral cutaneous nerve/lateral popliteal nerve*: The sensory loss is usually on the lateral aspect of the leg and dorsal surface of the foot. This nerve is commonly involved in leprosy and compressed at the head of the fibula. In India, individuals sit cross-legged for a prolonged period of time and if they have hereditary neuropathy with pressure palsies (HNPP) without realizing it, they may develop a lateral popliteal palsy with a foot drop and sensory loss. Subsequently in HNPP, the patient may give a positive family history of similar mononeuropathies in other family members.
  Note: In such cases, the ankle jerk is preserved; a point to help differentiate it from a L5–S1 root lesion due to a prolapsed intervertebral disc.
- *Sural nerve*: This nerve supplies a strip of skin below the lateral malleolus. Being a purely sensory nerve, a fascicular biopsy can be taken from this nerve without any significant sensory loss.
- *The medial and posterior tibial nerves*: These nerve supply the medial and lateral aspects, respectively, of the plantar surface of the foot. The integrity of the latter is important for eliciting the plantar response.

Mononeuropathy/Mononeuropathy Multiplex

In India, the most common etiology of mononeuropathy or MM will be leprosy **(Fig. 13.8)** closely followed by diabetes **(Box 13.5)**.

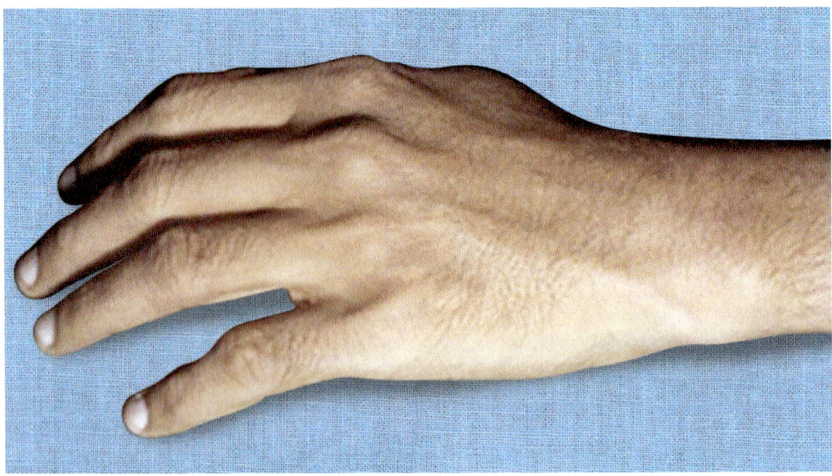

FIG. 13.8: Thickened distal cutaneous nerve with hypopigmented patch with hair loss in leprous neuritis.

BOX 13.5 | Etiologies of mononeuropathy multiplex.

- Leprosy
- Diabetes
- *Vasculitic*: Acute onset and painful
- MMN (pure motor) and MADSAM (motor/sensory)
- *Infections*: HIV, Lyme, herpes, and sarcoid (inflammation)
- Hereditary neuropathy with pressure palsy (HNPP)

[HIV: human immunodeficiency virus; MADSAM: multifocal-acquired demyelinating sensory and motor neuropathy; MMN: multifocal motor neuropathy (with conduction blocks)]

Disorders of Spinal Root

Involvement of the spinal roots also produces an asymmetrical loss of all the PSM.

In the ULs and LLs, dermatomes of the spinal roots are longitudinally oriented because of the growth of the limb buds and involve spinal segments C5–T1 and L1–S5. The maps of these spinal segments are also available in any textbook of clinical neurology. Over the trunk, the roots have a circular segmental orientation.

As mentioned earlier, there is a considerable overlap between two contiguous spinal roots. Hence, a clear-cut sensory demarcation is possible only if two or more spinal roots are involved. I would reiterate that a quicker and more appropriate response is elicited when one goes from an area of low sensitivity to an area of high sensitivity. For the above reasons, do not explore hypesthesia by going across contiguous roots. If, e.g., there is an area of hypesthesia over C5 (lateral aspect of the arm), then test the sensations over

C5 and immediately go and test the sensations over T1 (medial aspect of the arm). In the forearm and hand, test the medial versus the lateral aspect for quicker and more accurate results.

Similarly in the LLs, test the front of the thigh (L1, 2, 3) versus the back of the thigh (S2, 3), the medial (L4) versus the lateral part of the leg (L5). In the foot, the medial aspect is supplied by L5 whereas the lateral by S1.

Note that in the hand, the middle finger is C7 with C6 on the lateral side (index finger) and C8 on the medial side (ring and little fingers). In the posterior part of the leg, S2 is tucked between L4 and L5; so, go to the extreme medial and lateral part of the leg while testing L4 and L5, respectively, and stick more or less to the midline of the posterior part of the leg while testing for S2 sensory loss.

Differentiating between a mononeuropathy and a spinal root lesion is not difficult, as the areas of hypesthesia are distinctly dissimilar. Secondly, the muscles involved are much more in a root disorder. Lastly, the DTR are very useful in distinguishing one from the other. They are more likely to be absent in root lesions in comparison to mononeuropathies. For example, in a case of foot drop due to a lateral popliteal nerve palsy, the area of hypesthesia may be similar to that of L5. However, in a root lesion, the ankle jerk is absent (L5, S1) whereas it is preserved in a lateral popliteal nerve palsy.

PRIMARY SENSORY MODALITIES INVOLVED AT THE LEVEL OF THE SPINAL CORD

I will reiterate some anatomical facts which are important. The corticospinal tract (CST) has crossed before it descends in the spinal cord and is in the lateral white matter. Similarly, the STT has also crossed before it ascends in the anterolateral white matter. In contrast, the proprioceptive modalities (posterior column) ascend uncrossed. This gives rise to five patterns of PSM loss at the level of the spinal cord:

1. Involvement of all PSM below a clear-cut level occurs in a complete transection of the spinal cord and is adequately discussed in Chapter 12.
2. Involvement of the anterior part of the spinal cord due to an infarct in the anterior spinal artery territory. This involves the CST and the STTs in the lateral columns but spares posterior columns, hence so-called dissociation.
3. In a hemi-lesion of the spinal cord, the pyramidal and spinothalamic tracts are involved on one side and the proprioceptive modalities on the other—the Brown-Sequard syndrome.
4. In syringomyelia, axons of the second-order neurons for pain, temperature, and crude touch are involved in the anterior commissure as they cross over to the opposite side whereas the modality of light touch, which ascends uncrossed in the gracilis and cuneus fasciculus, is spared. In the affected area, pain and temperature are severely affected, but fine touch is spared—a true dissociate sensory loss.

5. Lastly, when the posterior columns (PC) are predominantly involved, the patient has a sensory ataxia. Two classic examples are B12 myelopathy and the "useless hand syndrome" due to compression of the PC by a meningioma/schwannoma at a high cervical cord level.

INVOLVEMENT OF THE PRIMARY SENSORY MODALITIES AT THE LEVEL OF THE BRAINSTEM

At the level of the brainstem, a "crossed dissociation" may occur. Here, the classic example is Wallenberg lateral medullary syndrome. The lesion involves the STT together with the neighboring sensory tract of the trigeminal nerve. Therefore, pain and temperature modalities are affected over the ipsilateral face and contralateral body. Again, light touch which ascends in the medial lemniscus is spared (see Fig. 12.5). The level of the brainstem is ascertained by the associated cranial nerve involvement.

INVOLVEMENT OF THE PRIMARY SENSORY MODALITIES AT THE LEVEL OF THE THALAMUS AND INTERNAL CAPSULE

A contralateral hemisensory deficit occurs if the thalamus or posterior limb of the IC is involved. Pure sensory strokes due to thalamic infarcts and hemorrhages are already covered in Chapter 12. In the IC, the sensory pathways are in the posterior third of the posterior limb. Lesions involving this area will produce a hemisensory deficit usually associated with hemiplegia. If the infarct is larger and extends posteriorly, it may involve the optic tracts producing, in addition, a homonymous hemianopia. Because of the crowding of the tracts, a small lesion produces severe deficits with a poor prognosis for good recovery.

RECOMMENDED ARTICLES

1. Campbell WW, Barohn RJ, Ranganathan LN. Cerebral sensory function. In: DeJong's The Neurological Examination, South Asian edition. New Delhi: Wolters Kluwer (India) Pvt Ltd; 2020. pp. 633-7.
2. Campbell WW, Barohn RJ, Ranganathan LN. Sensory localization. In DeJong's The Neurological Examination, South Asian edition. New Delhi: Wolters Kluwer (India) Pvt Ltd; 2020. pp. 639-54.
3. Davidoff RA, Spinal roots. In: Encyclopedia of Neurological Sciences. Amsterdam: Elsevier Science Inc; 2003. pp. 373-5.
4. Jewesbury ECO. Parietal lobe syndromes. In: Vinken PJ, Bruyn GW (Eds). Handbook of Clinical Neurology, volume 2. Amsterdam: North Holland Publishing Company; 1969. pp. 680-99.
5. Verhamme C, van Schaik IN. Polyneuropathies: Axonal. In: Hilton-Jones D, Turner MR (Eds). Oxford Textbook of Neuromuscular Disorders. New Delhi: Oxford University Press; 2015. pp. 132-42.

CHAPTER 14

Understanding Tone and Deep Tendon Reflexes

After an acute stroke or spinal cord lesion, there is initially flaccidity and areflexia, due to "shock" of the central nervous system (CNS). Only after a variable period do you initially get brisk and then exaggerated deep tendon reflexes (DTRs) followed by spasticity after another variable period. Why do brisk to exaggerated DTR precede spasticity? In order to understand this, one must understand the anatomy and physiology of the muscle spindle (MuS) and its role in the phasic stretch reflex (PSR) and tonic stretch reflex (TSR).

MUSCLE TONE

If a normal resting muscle is palpated, it possesses a certain amount of "tension." If it is passively stretched, there is some resistance to this stretching. This "tension" or "resistance" is called muscle tone. The muscle tone varies from muscle to muscle, being more in the antigravity muscles, particularly when adopting the vertical posture. Palpate your quadriceps muscle while sitting and then again in the standing position. The change in the muscle tone will be obvious to you.

The muscle tone is dependent on the function of the MuS, a spindle-shaped connective tissue capsule in which there are on an average 10 thin intrafusal muscle fibers (IFMF) **(Fig. 14.1)**. The MuS is very responsive to stretch and there is a high density of primary sensory nerve endings from the la thickly myelinated fibers, particularly in the equatorial area. The innervation of the IFMF comes from the gamma motor neurons (GMN) in the anterior horn of the spinal cord. Stimulation of the GMN produces a contraction of the IFMF, reducing the length of the MuS and keeping it in a "ready state," i.e., reducing the threshold for stimulation.

The GMN tone is influenced by several pathways, particularly the reticulospinal tract. This is the physiological basis of reinforcement in eliciting DTRs. When you ask a patient to try and pull apart his clasped hands, there is an increased sensory input into the reticular formation. This in turn increases descending impulses along the reticulospinal tract, thereby increasing GMN tone and keeping the MuS in a heightened state of contraction. Thus, the

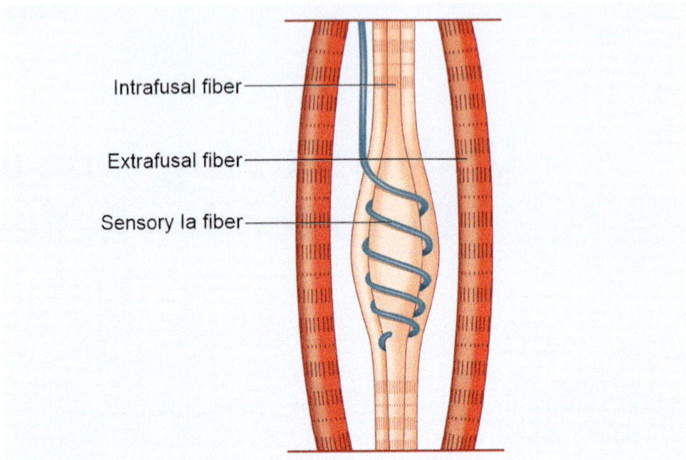

FIG. 14.1: Muscle spindle between two extrafusal fibers.

tendon reflex, which was originally sluggish, is better elicited. This is also the reason why highly anxious patients have brisk reflexes. In an upper motor neuron (UMN) lesion, the reticulospinal tracts are "free" of any inhibitory influences, thereby increasing the GMN tone and producing exaggerated DTR. Although the MuS is scattered throughout the muscle, the maximum density is at the origin and insertion of the muscle. The density of MuS also varies widely in different muscles. As a general rule, muscles used in delicate movements have a greater density than muscles which perform crude movements.

WHAT IS THE PHASIC AND TONIC STRETCH REFLEX?

The PSR is nothing but eliciting a DTR whereas the TSR is the passive contraction and lengthening of a muscle, an action that we do when testing the muscle tone at a joint. After an acute stroke or spinal cord lesion, there is initial flaccidity and areflexia due to "shock" of the nervous system. At this stage, there is no pyramidal or reticulospinal tone accounting for the flaccidity and areflexia. Only after a variable period is there a recovery of the reticulospinal and pyramidal tone. As both these systems recover, they are "free" from the inhibitory influences of the higher centers. Thus, you get initially exaggerated reflexes and subsequently spasticity. This implies that the PSR is a more sensitive parameter of a UMN pyramidal lesion and spasticity than the TSR. Let me clarify this statement by giving the example of the knee jerk after an acute stroke. When you tap the patellar tendon, there is a synchronous stretch of the IFMF of the MuS near the muscular area of the insertion of the quadriceps muscle. This produces a synchronous volley of excitatory impulses which travel very rapidly along the Ia thickly myelinated fibers to the spinal cord—the afferent arc of the knee jerk. These fibers have polysynaptic connections with the alpha motor neuron and produce a synchronous firing which travels along the efferent arc to the motor nerve innervation of the quadriceps muscle, thereby producing a brisk contraction of the muscle. On the other hand, passive stretching of the muscles, as we do when testing the tone, produces asynchronous stretching of the MuS scattered all along the muscle. This results in an asynchronous volley of impulses going along the afferent arc and asynchronously firing the alpha motor neurons. This asynchronous contraction of the extrafusal muscle fibers of the quadriceps muscle scattered throughout the muscle is not of sufficient threshold to detect spasticity. Thus, PSR is a more sensitive index of spasticity than TSR. The corollary to this statement is that when there is spasticity, the DTR have to be exaggerated unless there is a concurrent lower motor neuron (LMN) lesion.

The localizing value of the DTR lies in the absence of the reflex. Let me clarify with an example. In a case of viral transverse myelitis, the lesion is never truly transverse. In the acute phase, there is an area of edema surrounding the core area of involvement. If the core lesion is at C7, edema will extend for one to two segments above and below it. Edema in the segment above may give rise to a brisk biceps jerk after a variable period. That does not mean that the localization of the lesion is above C5–6. The lesion is at the level of the absent DTR, in this case, an absent triceps jerk (C7) **(Table 14.1)**.

TABLE 14.1: Root value and the nerves involved in the DTRs.

Jerk	Root value	Nerve
Biceps	C5–6	Musculocutaneous
Supinator	C5–6	Radial
Triceps	C6–7	Radial
Knee	L2, 3, 4	Femoral
Ankle	S1	Posterior tibial

Another tip that I can give you is that in some situations, you "titrate" a DTR. When you see a patient with residual ischemic neurological deficit for a follow-up, there is hardly any objective evidence of the stroke. This is the situation in which I like to titrate the DTR, which is very eloquently done with the knee jerk. Bend both the knees and keep the patellar tendons side by side. Then start tapping each tendon lightly and more lightly with each tap until you are able to elicit the reflex only on one side. In this way, you can objectively establish the affected side.

Lastly, while I am on the topic of the DTR, I would like to comment on the plantar response (L5, S1). Many patients at JJ Hospital had extremely calloused feet as shown in **Figure 14.2A**. In one such patient, I, as a house officer, found it impossible to elicit his plantar response. On the next day, while on the rounds, Dr BS Singhal asked me about the patient's plantar response. I frankly told him that I was unable to elicit the plantar response. He gave me a wry smile, picked up a tuning fork, and elicited the plantar response with its working end. Ever since that day, I have used my tuning fork to elicit plantar responses in patients with calloused feet **(Figs. 14.2A to C)**.

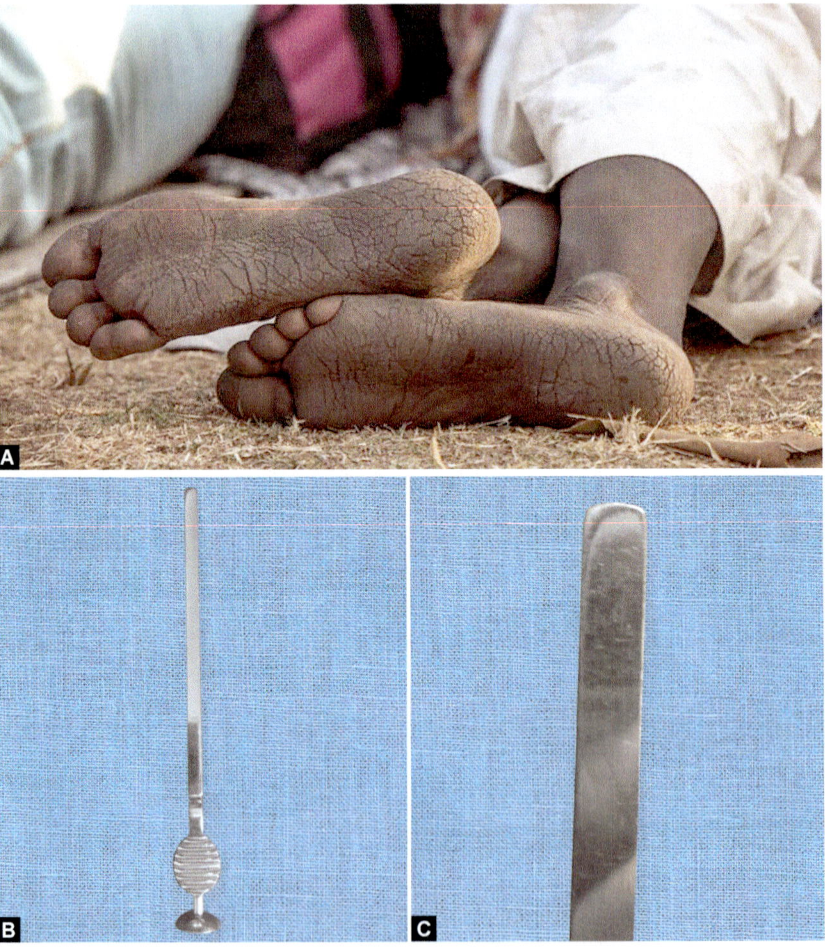

FIGS. 14.2A TO C: (A) Calloused feet; (B) My tuning fork; (C) Enlarge view of my tuning fork. Note the worn-out edge after years of eliciting the plantar response.

The change in muscle tone in pathological states is either hypertonia in UMN states or hypotonia in LMN states. In UMN states, there is spasticity in pyramidal tract lesions as already explained and rigidity in extrapyramidal disorders. The latter is beyond the scope of this book. In LMN states, the extrafusal muscle fibers (EFMF) as well as the IFMF are denervated, hence the hypotonia.

RECOMMENDED ARTICLE

1. Brodal A (Ed). The peripheral motor neurone. In: Neurological Anatomy: In Relation to Clinical Medicine. New York: Oxford University Press; 1969. pp. 117-150.

CHAPTER 15

Altered State of Consciousness: Clinical Assessment of Stupor and Coma in the Intensive Care Unit

I have written a complete chapter on this topic. Here, I would like to stress on a few "birdsongs" to remember during the clinical assessment of a patient with deteriorating level of consciousness (LOC).

- When the central nervous system (CNS) is affected by the disease process, the LOC deteriorates. This can range from hypersomnia, at one end of the spectrum, to coma at the other end. This deterioration is assessed by two parameters: Alertness and awareness. Thus, the patient may be:
  - Alert and aware—normal state
  - Alert but not aware—acute confusional state, delirium, akinetic mutism, minimally conscious state (MCS), and persistent vegetative state (PVS)
  - Not alert and not aware—stupor and coma

  There is only one exception to this rule. In the "locked-in state", the patient is alert and aware but is paralyzed below the level of the eyes.
- The etiologies of coma are many. As a general rule, it requires a large hemispheric lesion or a small discreet rostral brainstem lesion (above the upper two-third of the pons) to produce coma. In the former, stupor and coma result from edema and subsequent coning. In the latter, the small discreet lesion involves the ascending reticular activating system. There are early abnormalities of the external ocular movements (EOM) and oculocephalic maneuvers (OCM)/oculovestibular reflex (OVR) because of the proximity of the pathways, particularly the medial longitudinal fasciculus (MLF), subserving these functions or reflexes, to the ascending reticular activating system.
- Physicians must also be aware of depression of the brainstem by drugs or toxins. These drugs and toxins preferentially "knock out" the MLF. Brainstem depression is suspected when the pupillary response and the corneal reflexes are preserved out of proportion to the OCM/OVR because the latter are only elicited if the MLF is functional. When brainstem depression is suspected because of the above features, it may be confirmed by irrigating one ear with ice cold water. This produces upward deviation of the eyes, instead of horizontal deviation which would only be possible if the MLF was functional.

- A standard neurological examination is not applicable to a patient of stupor/coma. Neurological examination of such patients is limited and involves judging reflex activity.
  - Always rule out fracture of the cervical spine or skull base before checking out for neck stiffness. In such cases, the "Battle sign" is useful for occult skull base fractures **(Fig. 15.1)**.
  - The fundus is checked for evidence of hypertension or diabetes. Do not forget that a subhyaloid hemorrhage is practically diagnostic of a subarachnoid hemorrhage (SAH) **(Fig. 15.2)**.

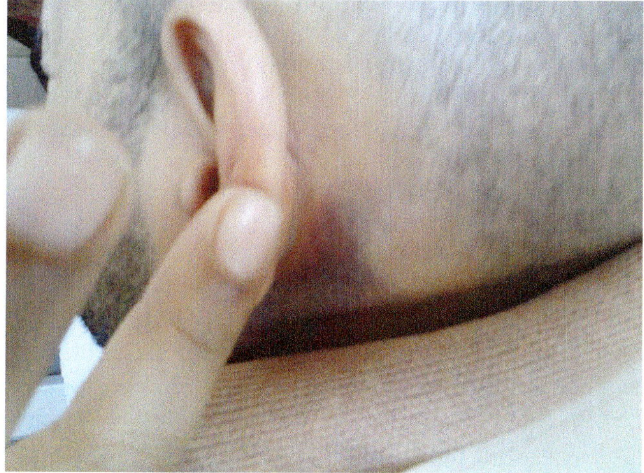

FIG. 15.1: Battle sign. Note ecchymosis behind the ear and at the tip of the mastoid.

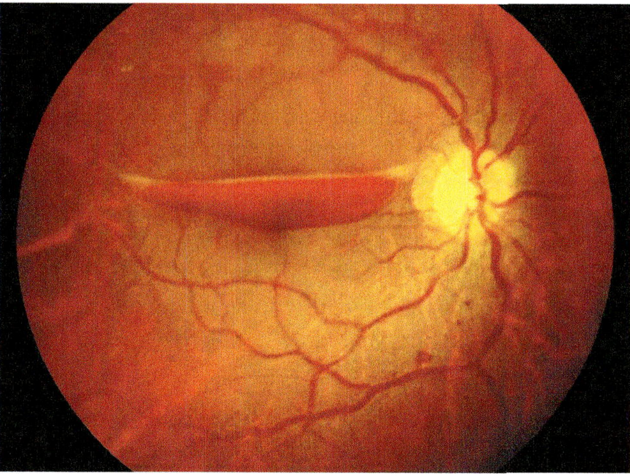

FIG. 15.2: Fundal photograph showing a subhyaloid hemorrhage.
Courtesy: Dr Phiroze Patel.

- There are a few simple observations of the patient which give good motor or lateralizing signs: Weakness, unilateral grasp reflex, and focal clonic or myoclonic seizure activity establish the abnormal side.
- In an agitated patient, who is plucking or clutching at his clothes, the corticospinal tracts are intact. Similarly, grimacing to deep supraorbital painful stimulus indicates that the corticobulbar tracts up to the pons are intact.
- Spontaneous roving eye movements indicate an intact pons, MLF, and midbrain as these structures are involved in conjugate roving eye movements.
- Multifocal myoclonus is seen in hypoxic ischemic encephalopathy (HIE) and indicates a poor prognosis for meaningful neurological recovery. Lastly, orofacial dyskinesias are seen in metabolic encephalopathy.

- Once a neurological examination is done, classify the comatose patient into three groups:
  1. Coma with focal signs—strokes, tumors
  2. Coma without focal but with meningeal signs:
     - With fever—encephalitis, meningitis
     - Without fever—SAH
  3. Coma without focal and meningeal signs—hypoxic-ischemic encephalopathy (HIE), metabolic/toxic encephalopathy

  Note: In the real world, there may be overlaps between these groups. In a case of SAH, initially the patient may fit into coma without focal but with meningeal signs. Subsequently, the patient may develop fever because of blood in the CSF and also focal signs as a late complication of vasospasm. Hence, this classification is applicable when you examine the patient during the acute phase of the coma.
- Please remember that in a patient in the intensive care unit (ICU), any sudden and unexplained change in the LoC warrants an urgent EEG to rule out nonconvulsive status epilepticus (NCSE).

  Case vignette: NSB, 72-year-old female patient with chronic kidney disease, was on injection Cefotaxime for urinary tract infection. Her husband, who was a consultant orthopedic surgeon, was chatting with her and then wished her good night before leaving. He suddenly noticed that she was unresponsive and informed the emergency doctor. An EEG, done on January 5, 2008, showed NCSE **(Fig. 15.3A)**. She was given the necessary antiseizure therapy and recovered completely. A repeat EEG showed only nonspecific slowing (drug-induced drowsiness) **(Fig. 15.3B)**.

- Also remember that the antibiotics commonly used in the ICU have many adverse effects which involve the nervous system. These side effects are particularly seen in elderly patients, in chronic kidney disease, in patients with prior CNS disease, and for metronidazole in patients with

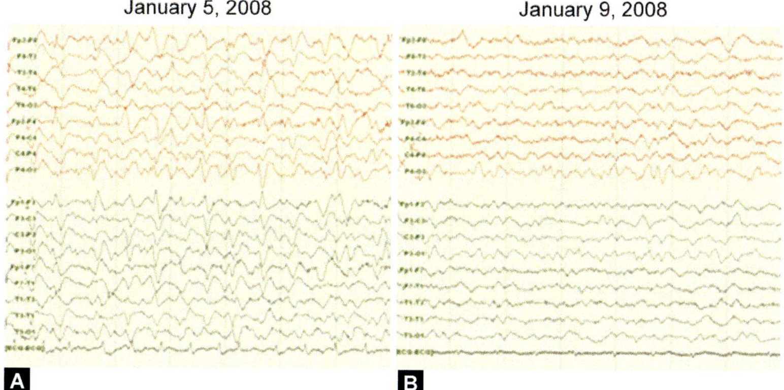

FIGS. 15.3A AND B: (A) EEG of January 5, 2008, suggestive of NCSE; (B) EEG of January 9, 2008, control of NCSE.
(NCSE: nonconvulsive status epilepticus)

chronic liver disease. Most importantly, one must realize that Cefepime can produce a coma. This evolves after 1–10 days of administration and takes 2–7 days to resolve. Lack of awareness of this adverse effect may lead to many unnecessary investigations and at times a disastrous outcome. Therefore, it is a good practice to go through the drug regimen that the patient is getting.

- Lastly, the outcome of coma is dependent on a combination of the etiology, severity, and duration, the presence or absence of the pupillary response, corneal reflex, OCM/OVR at 24 hours, and the motor response to pain. Prognosis is therefore best judged at 24 hours after the initial assessment. Also remember that there are two physical findings that carry a good prognosis for recovery: (1) the presence of nystagmus and (2) grimacing of the face when you give a painful supraorbital stimulus. The former indicates that the saccadic component has returned reflecting a reversible dysfunction of the parapontine reticular formation (PPRF). The latter, as already mentioned, indicates intact corticobulbar tracts up to the facial nucleus in the pons.

RECOMMENDED ARTICLES

1. Bates D. Coma. In: Swash M, Oxbury J (Eds), Clinical Neurology. London: Churchill Livingston Publishers; 1991; pp. 188-204.
2. Grill MF, Maganti RK. Neurotoxic effects associated with antibiotic use: management considerations. Br J Clin Pharmacol. 2011;72:381-93.
3. Katrak SM. Coma in the ICU: A Clinical Approach. In: Khadilkar SV, Singh G (Eds), IAN Textbook of Neurology, 2nd edition. New Delhi: Jaypee Brothers Medical Publishers; 2024. pp. 248-52.

CHAPTER 16

A Simplified Understanding of the Neurogenic Bladder

One of the "blind spots" that I had in neurology was the understanding of the neurogenic bladder. Therefore, in May 2020, I made a concerted effort to understand the function of the urinary bladder in health and disease. The best way for me is to prepare a teaching power-point lecture. Only if I understand the working of the urinary bladder could I impart it to the students. In this chapter, I have drawn heavily from the publications of Professor Claire Fowler and her team from the Uro-Neurology Unit at the National Hospital of Neurology and Neurosurgery, University College London, Queen's Square, London, UK.

Simply put, the main function of the bladder is storage of urine and voiding. If one takes 2–3 minutes to void and do so four to five times a day, depending on the weather and hydration, over 95% of our lifetime, the bladder serves to store urine. The bladder cannot store urine indefinitely and at some stage there is a "phasic switching" from storage to voiding. This switch is under voluntary control: A unique feature of the bladder which sets it apart from the other autonomically controlled organs like the heart and blood vessels. During storage, the detrusor is relaxed and the sphincters are contracted and during voiding, the reverse happens, i.e., the detrusor contracts and the sphincters relax. This voluntary switch is controlled by a complex neural network involving higher cortical centers in the forebrain and certain centers in the pons. Thus, the term "neurogenic bladder" denotes lower urinary tract (LUT) dysfunction caused by malfunctioning of these "switching control centers," besides disorders involving the spinal cord, cauda equina, and peripheral innervation of the bladder.

Autonomic Innervation of the Bladder (Fig. 16.1)

The sympathetic innervation arises from T11 to L2 and via the inferior mesenteric and superior hypogastric plexus forms the hypogastric nerve. β-adrenergic receptors are inhibitory to the detrusor and α-1 adrenergic receptors are excitatory to the internal sphincter (IS).

The parasympathetic innervation arises from S2 to S4 and via the pelvic plexus forms the pelvic nerves, which innervate the detrusor. The M3

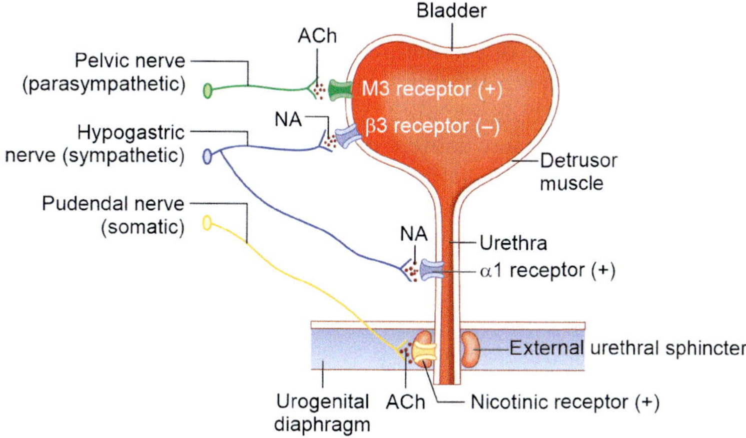

FIG. 16.1: Autonomic and somatic innervations of the bladder.
[ACh: acetylcholine; α1: adrenergic receptor; β3: adrenergic receptors; M3: muscarinic 3 cholinergic receptors; NA: noradrenaline; (+): excitatory; (-): inhibitory]

acetylcholine receptors are excitatory to the detrusor. During voiding, there is increased parasympathetic tone, with contraction of the detrusor and reciprocal relaxation of the IS because of suppressed sympathetic tone.

The somatic innervation arises from S2 to S4 and forms the pudendal nerve which innervates the striated fibers of the external sphincter. Acetylcholine-N receptors are excitatory to the external sphincter.

Afferent Innervation

The sensation of filling is conveyed by the Aδ fibers, via the hypogastric (body and bladder neck), pelvic (only body), and pudendal (urethra) nerves. These afferent impulses ascend and via the dorsal root ganglion of T11-L2 and S2-S4 enter the spinal cord and project directly to the midbrain periaqueductal gray (PAG).

As mentioned earlier, bladder filling is not indefinite; the bladder must empty at some stage. This "switching" is under voluntary control. This voluntary switching is dependent on two aspects: Mechanical and social.

Mechanical aspect: As the bladder fills, the Aδ fiber-mediated afferent signals increase in frequency and intensity. The individual gets an initial sensation of filling and, with time, a sensation to void. The latter then becomes a strong sensation to void and if appropriate circumstances are not prevalent, it can lead to urge incontinence, particularly in the elderly. Thus, the first aspect of voluntary switching is dependent on the amount of urine in the bladder—is there enough urine in the bladder to void!

Social aspect: As the individual gets a strong sensation to void, the social aspect kicks in. Simply put, is it socially appropriate to void? Is there a toilet nearby and is it vacant? I am very fond of a saying, "How long a minute is, depends on which side of the bathroom door you are on". This aspect of social appropriateness was beautifully portrayed by Peter Sellers in the film "The Party". Lastly, in countries where open air voiding is prevalent, a "safe" situation may also come into contention.

This mechanical and social appropriateness is very succinctly termed "safe-to-void" or "unsafe-to-void" by the uro-neurology group, Queen's Square, and is governed by three important areas—the midbrain PAG, the pontine micturition center (PMC), and several areas in the forebrain, which I like to collectively call the higher neural control of micturition (HNC).

The Midbrain Periaqueductal Grey

The midbrain PAG is the rostral terminus of the afferent signals of bladder filling from the Aδ fibers. The PAG constantly distributes the frequency and intensity of these signals to several areas in the forebrain. There are feedback signals from these areas to the PAG, regarding appropriateness to void. The PAG in turn has a tonic suppressive effect on the PMC and based on inputs from the HNC either continues this tonic suppression or releases the PMC from it.

Pontine Micturition Center

Functional magnetic resonance imaging (MRI) studies have identified a medial and a lateral pontine PMC (mPMC and ltPMC). Activation of the mPMC promotes voiding by sharply increasing the intravesicular pressure and relaxing the sphincters. On the other hand, activation of the ltPMC promotes continence by increasing the contraction of the sphincters. The activation of either the medial or the lateral PMC is through signals received from the PAG as the PMC has no direct afferents from the bladder.

Higher Neural Control of Micturition

In the forebrain, there are many areas involved in the HNC of micturition. Collectively, they are responsible for the voluntary switching from storage to voiding. In each individual, there is a certain "default" setting for voiding. The main question is, "when to switch?" The centers in the forebrain collate the data provided by the PAG and answer this question! The main areas involved in the HNC of micturition are the dorsal anterior cingulate gyrus (dACC) and the insula in conjunction with the lateral prefrontal cortex (ltPFC) and the medial prefontal cortex (mPFC). These areas do not function in isolation but interact with each other and receive inputs from the supplementary motor area, parahippocampal gyrus, and hypothalamus.

The dACC is the so-called autonomic motor cortex. It generates the desire to void and the reaction to it, i.e., to postpone voiding or not. It can judge the emotional appropriateness, i.e., whether there is a subtle difference between "a strong desire to void" and "urgency." The dACC has the capacity to differentiate this subtle difference in order to postpone or initiate voiding. The insula and the ltPFC are the so-called autonomic sensory cortex. The insula interacts with the ltPFC and judges the qualitative value of bladder filling: Is the sensation comfortable, tolerable, or uncomfortable? The mPFC is the seat for appropriate social behavior and plans the appropriateness of micturition. It is involved when a voluntary decision about voiding is required and therefore has a strong direct influence on the PAG either maintaining or deactivating the tonic suppression.

Hence, the sequence of events in normal continence and voiding is shown in **Figures 16.2 and 16.3**.

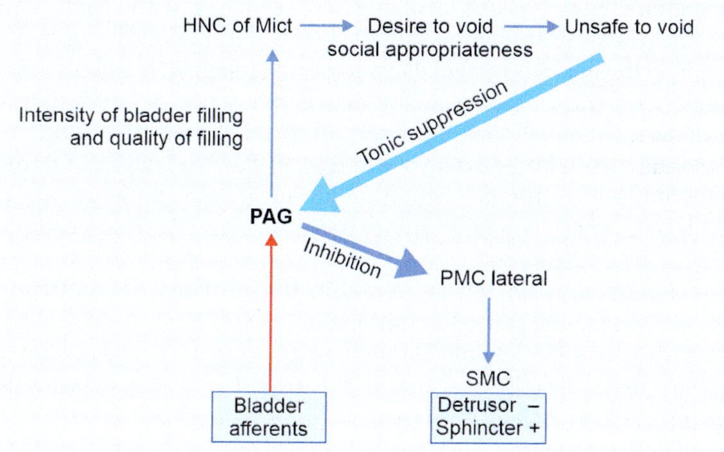

FIG.16.2: Circuit to maintain continence.

(HNC of Mict: higher neural control of micturition; PAG: periaqueductal gray; PMC: pontine micturition center; SMC: sacral micturition center; +: contracting; –: relaxation)

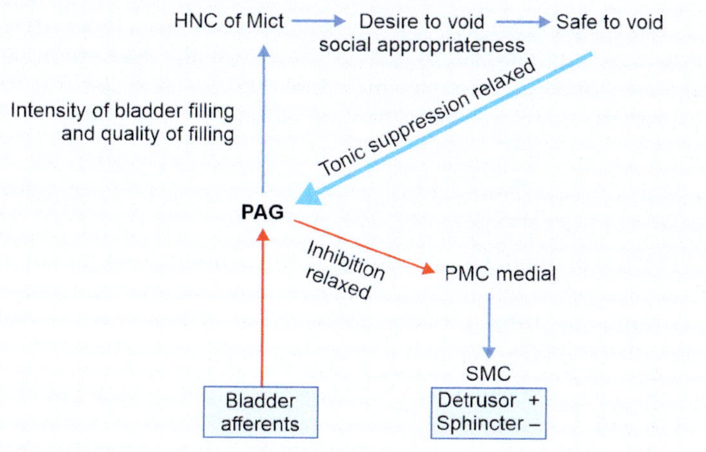

FIG. 16.3: Circuit for voluntary switch to voiding.

(HNC of Mict: higher neural control of micturition; PAG: periaqueductal gray; PMC: pontine micturition center; SMC: sacral micturition center; +: contracting; –: relaxation)

Thus, LUT dysfunction can occur at:

- *Suprapontine level*: Frontal lobe, basal ganglia, and midbrain level
- *Pontine level*: Rare
- *Spinal cord level*: Particularly lumbosacral cord
- *Cauda equina level*: Very early LUT dysfunction
- *Peripheral innervation*: Uncommon

Symptoms and signs will depend on the site of involvement and may involve purely upper motor neuron (UMN) signs (suprapontine problems), pure lower motor neuron signs (cauda equina/peripheral innervation), or a combination of both (lesions involving lower spinal cord and cauda equina). Hence, the clinical examination should be directed at establishing the level of the lesion in the nervous system. Do not rely too much on bladder symptoms. Frequency, urgency, or urge incontinence can occur in any lesion above the lumbosacral spinal cord. However, in a spinal cord lesion, the patient has incontinence with awareness whereas in the late stages of dementia, the patient has incontinence without awareness. Some patients with cauda equina lesions and secondary urinary tract infection (UTI) may complain of urgency in the early stages.

One should, however, rely on a combination of symptoms and signs. In a spinal cord lesion, one can get a combination of LUT and sexual dysfunction, whereas with an enlarged prostate there will be only LUT dysfunction. I may stress here that a history of sexual dysfunction is grossly neglected in our clinical practice, especially in women.

Another two aspects of an extended clinical evaluation of a patient with a neurogenic bladder are worth mentioning:

Postvoid residue (PVR): The history of incomplete voiding is usually not a reliable index of a PVR. The PVR can be reliably assessed on the ultrasound sonography (USG) or a quick "in-and-out-catheterization." Any PVR of >100 mL has the potential of a UTI and the patient should be advised clean intermittent self-catheterization (CISC). This is usually the case in patients with infrasacral lesions. Patients with spinal cord problems have a PVR but usually <100 mL. They may be monitored closely on anticholinergic drugs. Patients with suprapontine lesions are incontinent without any PVR.

Neurological per-rectal (PR) examination: The anal tone is a good reflection of the state of the external sphincter as they share a common motor innervation: S2 to S4 and the pudendal nerve. However, the neurological PR examination should only be performed in cases of cauda equina or peripheral innervation problems. After inserting your index finger in the anal canal, ask the patient, "what would you do if you had a strong urge to pass stool and you did not want to dirty your clothes?" He or she will contract the anal sphincter. Judge the "power" around your index finger. Normally, it is a tight squeeze and is easily differentiated from a weak anal sphincter. If there is total denervation, the anal sphincter is patulous and there is no "resistance" to the entry of your index finger.

The most common suprapontine lesions are (1) frontal lobe lesions, (2) multiple system atrophy-parkinsonian type (MSA-P), and (3) Parkinson's disease (PD).

Frontal lobe lesions: In such lesions, the bladder dysfunction is because of lack of inhibition of the PAG and thus the PMC. There is socially inappropriate voiding with associated neuropsychiatric symptoms and signs. In the early stages, there maybe awareness of incontinence but in the late stages the patient is not aware. As mentioned earlier, there is no PVR. The main etiologies are traumatic brain injury (TBI), strokes, dementias [Alzheimer's disease (AD) and frontotemporal dementia (FTD)], normal pressure hydrocephalus (NPH), advanced multiple sclerosis (MS), and frontal lobe gliomas.

MSA-P: The earliest features are erectile dysfunction followed later by urgency and urge incontinence. If both occur early, the prognosis is poor. Initially, there is detrusor overactivity but as the disease progresses there is voiding dysfunction with detrusor inactivity. Thus, there is incomplete voiding and an increasing PVR, a feature characteristic of MSA-P. Thus, follow-up USG assessment of PVR helps to differentiate it from PD. In the late stages, because of the involvement of the sympathetic innervation, there is incontinence with a lax IS. The external sphincter is also involved because of loss of neurons in Onuf's nucleus in the sacral spinal cord.

PD: In PD, the main autonomic problem is constipation. Urinary complaints do occur but late in the disease. There is detrusor overactivity with nocturia and urgency in the majority of patients. Unlike MSA-P, the PVR is typically low.

Pontine lesions: As brainstem lesions produce a lot of signs, isolated bladder dysfunction in pontine lesions is very uncommon. Rarely discrete lesions in the tectal area of the midbrain may produce bladder dysfunction by affecting the PAG.

Spinal cord lesions: In the spinal cord, bladder dysfunction is early and more severe in lesions of the lumbosacral area. In the thoracic area, symptoms occur pari passu with the paralytic signs. In the high cervical area, usually compression, I have rarely seen bladder involvement. At the JJ Hospital, we had many patients who were quadriparetic from atlantoaxial dislocation, but none of them had bladder involvement.

Bladder involvement is more common in acute involvements of the spinal cord, be it trauma or acute compression from a pathological vertebral collapse. Initially, there is spinal shock with retention of urine which will need catheterization. The retention should be detected early. I have seen many patients with an overdistended bladder and overflow incontinence. On catheterization, between 700 and 1,000 cc of urine is drained. The net result is that the detrusor is overstretched and on recovery, there is detrusor underactivity. A rule of the thumb states that with 1 hour of retention, the bladder will take 24 hours to recover and beyond a certain point in time, it is unlikely that there will be any recovery. Hence, in the acute stages, palpating or percussing (unfortunately a lost art) for a full bladder is imperative. With a severe lesion, voiding becomes a segmental reflex—the so-called automatic bladder **(Figs. 16.4A and B)**. In health, unmyelinated afferent c-fibers are unimportant in generating detrusor contractions, as the Aδ fibers directly convey the relevant information to the PAG. With a severe spinal cord lesion, the circuit involving Aδ fibers is nonfunctional; so the c-fibers become the main afferent arc for detrusor contraction. This segmental reflex gives rise to detrusor overactivity which is ill sustained and weak. Besides this, it must be noted that the PMC controls the reciprocal activity of the detrusor and sphincters. When the PMC is "disconnected", you get weak, ill-sustained detrusor activity against uncoordinated sphincters—detrusor-sphincter dyssynergia (DSD). The net result is incomplete voiding, increasing PVR, LUT infections, and intermittent increase in intravesical pressure (detrusor contraction against uncoordinated closed sphincters). This in turn increases the risk of upper UTI and renal failure. Both the detrusor overactivity and DSD correlate with the duration and extent of the pyramidal damage.

Cauda equina lesions: In a cauda equina problem, both the afferent sensory inputs and the efferent motor innervations of the bladder are involved. Urinary retention is the most common presenting symptom associated with fecal incontinence. As the sensory afferents are affected, there is no urge to urinate, and overflow incontinence follows. Spontaneous detrusor contractions are lacking, and low-level weak detrusor overactivity persists. As the sphincters are also weak, this results in constant dribbling of urine. The PVR is usually high (over 100 mL). The clinical features may vary depending

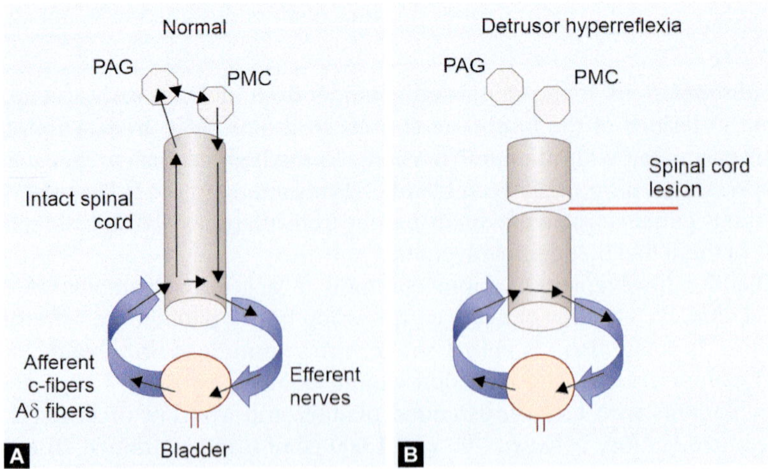

FIGS.16.4A AND B: Circuit for a segmental reflex in a suprasacral spinal cord lesion. (PAG: periaqueductal gray; PMC: pontine micturition center)

on whether the onset is acute or gradual. If the etiology is an acute intervertebral disc prolapse or tuberculosis spinal meningitis, the patient may have acute low backache and bilateral but asymmetrical root pains. Weakness of the lower limbs is also asymmetrical and distal more than proximal. The sensory loss is usually along the posterior aspect of the thigh (S2-3) and perianal region (S3-5)—the classic saddle anesthesia. The anal sphincter tone is weak or lost, explaining the associated fecal incontinence. In males, sexual dysfunction involves erection and lack of ejaculation whereas in females, it involves absence of orgasm and vaginal lubrication.

An acute cauda equina syndrome is a medical emergency. The retention of urine should be detected early and the patient catheterized, to prevent massive retention with overflow incontinence. The next step is to establish the etiology and start appropriate therapy. If the etiology is an acute disc prolapse, emergency decompression will go a long way in improving bladder, bowel, and sexual dysfunction. For residual bladder dysfunction, CISC, three to four times a day, is preferred to avoid long-term catheterization and UTI.

Lesions of the peripheral innervation: This usually implies peripheral neuropathy. It must be remembered that the bladder innervation is over a short length of nerve fibers. Therefore, in length-dependent peripheral neuropathies, like diabetes, the bladder involvement is late with well-established symptoms and signs of a peripheral neuropathy. In diabetic bladder dysfunction, the sensory afferents are more affected, resulting in a large capacity bladder. It is not unusual to have 700 mL of urine on USG before the first urge to void occurs. Detrusor contractions do occur but are weaker than normal, resulting in a high PVR. Secondly, orthostatic hypotension and male erectile dysfunction occur earlier than bladder dysfunction. In fact, erectile dysfunction may be the presenting symptom in some cases of unsuspected diabetes.

THERAPY OF THE NEUROGENIC BLADDER

I will outline the principles of therapy together with some details of the therapy of an overactive bladder (OAB).

The main aim of therapy is to achieve urinary continence, thereby preventing UTI, preserving upper urinary tract function, and, very importantly, improving the quality of life for the individual. Therapy, in a hierarchal fashion, involves conservative measures, nonsurgical and then surgical interventions.

Conservative measures involve bladder training and pharmacotherapy. Nonsurgical interventions are intravesicular botulinum toxin injections, particularly in cases of spinal cord trauma and MS and percutaneous posterior tibial nerve stimulation. The posterior tibial nerve is the large terminal branch of the sciatic nerve with a root value of L4-5 S1-3. Lastly, surgical interventions are sacral nerve neuromodulation, bladder augmentation, anterior root stimulation, and continent/incontinent diversion.

Bladder training: This is effective in incontinence due to cognitive and motor deficits, i.e., OAB. One of the important steps is to maintain a bladder diary. This helps in establishing a realistic voiding interval and then instructing the patient in doing timed voiding. Fluid intake, reducing caffeine/alcohol, and avoiding diuretic therapy are other measures which help maintaining continence. Biofeedback pelvic floor muscle training is useful in cases of stress incontinence, particularly in multiparous females. It suppresses activity in the dACC and reduces the fear of incontinence.

Pharmacotherapy for LUT dysfunction should be individualized based on the degree of bother to the patient, medication side-effect profile, concomitant comorbidities, and current medication regimen, particularly for drugs with anticholinergic side effects.

The bladder may be OAB or underactive bladder (UAB). In OAB, the main receptors which are targeted are (1) antimuscarinic cholinergic receptors and (2) β-adrenergic receptor agonist. Other drugs that are used are imipramine, a tricyclic antidepressant medication, and the benzodiazepines (See **Fig. 16.1**, page 125).

There is no effective therapy for a UAB, but some medications have been used with limited success—muscarinic receptor agonists to increase the detrusor tone, anticholinesterase inhibitors again to increase acetylcholine levels and thereby increase detrusor tone, and α-adrenergic receptor antagonists to relax the IS **(See Fig. 16.1)**.

The bladder may also be involved at the level of the outlet. Decreased resistance of the outlet results in stress incontinence. This is best managed with biofeedback pelvic floor muscle training together with an α-adrenergic receptor agonist to increase the IS tone and/or β-adrenergic receptor agonist to reduce detrusor contractions and/or imipramine. Increased resistance at the outlet results in bladder outflow obstruction. This is managed by α-adrenergic receptor antagonists, to relax the IS, together with benzodiazepines, baclofen, or phosphodiesterase inhibitors.

Anticholinergic therapy for OAB **(Table 16.1)**: Anticholinergic drugs (AChD) block the muscarinic (M3) cholinergic receptors at the detrusor muscle, thus decreasing detrusor overactivity. But no drug is totally selective for the detrusor and therefore acts at other muscarinic sites to produce side effects—dry mouth and eyes, constipation, confusion in the elderly, blurred vision, somnolence, and tachycardia. The newer AChDs have similar efficacy but have a greater bladder selectivity, thereby reducing side effects. Hence, the choice of an AChD is not based on efficacy but on the side-effect profile.

Oxybutynin is considered the first-line drug because of its cost effectiveness, safety, efficacy, and tolerability in a considerable proportion of patients. Start therapy at a low dose, 2.5 mg BID, and then gradually increase the dose to a maximum of 5 mg TID if the PVR < 100 mL. Monitor the PVR every 2 weeks to judge the efficacy of therapy. Oxybutynin with bladder training results in a good outcome at the lowest possible dose. If the side effects are

TABLE 16.1: Frequently used anticholinergic drugs.

Name	Receptor selectivity	Central nervous system levels*	Other side effects
Oxybutynin	Nonselective	Mod/High	Mod/High
Tolterodine	Nonselective	Low	50% of oxybutynin
Solifenacin	M2, M3	Low	Low rate
Darifenacin	M3	Low	Low rate
Trospium	Nonselective	Very low	Low rate
Fesoterodine	Nonselective	Low	Low rate

*CNS levels reflect the drug's ability to cross the blood–brain barrier.
(M2: muscarinic 2 receptors; M3: muscarinic 3 receptors)

unmanageable, switch to a second-line drug like tolterodine and monitor the PVR. The patient may be referred for specialized care in case of failure to respond to second-line drug therapy. In spinal cord lesions with DSD, AChDs with judicious use of CISC are very effective. Before starting AChDs, it is important to document the current regimen of drugs that the patient is on, particularly for drugs with high anticholinergic action. This is essential as drug interaction may result in adverse side effects and discontinuation of anticholinergics for the OAB.

β-3 receptor agonists (BRAg) are the newer groups of drugs used for OAB—mirabegron and vibegron. β-3 receptor activation produces detrusor relaxation, thus resulting in their use for OAB. Mirabegron can be synergistically combined with Solifenacin. They produce a lesser degree of dry mouth and constipation. BRAgs must be used cautiously (mirabegron > vibegron) in patients with concomitant ischemic heart disease as their serious side effects include rise of BP, tachycardia, and atrial fibrillation. Mirabegron is contraindicated in patients with severe uncontrolled hypertension.

I hope this simplified explanation of the normal functioning of the urinary bladder helped you to understand the complex neural control involved in maintaining continence. Once that is understood, it becomes easier to understand the dysfunctions of the bladder from lesions at various levels of the neural pathways. I would like to reiterate the importance of the PVR not only in making decisions for management but also in monitoring the efficacy of drug therapy. The principles of pharmacotherapy for an OAB have been explained.

RECOMMENDED ARTICLES

1. Fowler CJ. Neurological disorders of micturition and their treatment. Brain. 1999;122:1213-31.
2. Fowler CJ, Dalton C, Panicker JN. Review of neurologic diseases for the urologist. Urol Clin N Am. 2010;37:517-26.

3. Fowler CJ, Griffiths D, de Groat WC. The neural control of micturition. Nat Rev Neurosci. 2008;9:453-66.
4. Griffiths D. Neural control of micturition in humans: a working model. Nat Rev Neurosci. 2015;12(12):695-705.
5. Kuteesa W, Moore KH. Anticholinergic drugs for overactive bladder. Aust Prescr. 2006;29:22-4.
6. Panicker JN. Urogenital symptoms in neurologic patients. Continuum. 2017;23:533-52.
7. Panicker JN. Fowler CJ. The bare essentials: uro-neurology. Pract Neurol. 2010;10: 178-85.
8. Panicker JN, de Sèze, Fowler CJ. Neurogenic lower urinary tract dysfunction and its management. Clin Rehab. 2010;4:579-89.

CHAPTER 17

Some of My Statements with Meaning

- ***"If you have more than three differential diagnoses you do not know what you are treating"***.
  During an interview, the legendary neurologist Professor Raymond Adams said, "a long list of differential diagnoses is in fact a failed diagnosis". A long list of differential diagnosis denotes that you have good theoretical knowledge but cannot apply it in practical terms. I prefer a very compact list of differential diagnosis and hence my statement to my postgraduate students.
- ***"Common things occur commonly"***.
  I frequently make this statement when neurosarcoidosis is placed above central nervous system (CNS) tuberculosis (TB) in the differential diagnosis. I emphasize that commonly occurring "large print" diagnosis should come way before uncommon or rarely seen "fine print" entities. This is also true for the postgraduates' favorite diagnosis of paraneoplastic syndromes.
- ***"In the shadow of diabetes is TB"***.
  This statement is true for India where both diabetes and TB are common. When dealing with a case of suspected meningitis in a patient with diabetes, keep this statement in mind.
- ***"Peripheral nerves tingle, Roots pain"***.
  When the history points to a problem in the peripheral nervous system, pay heed to this statement. The exception to this statement is in painful peripheral neuropathies where pain is a dominant presenting symptom (see Box 13.2 on page 108).
- ***"Peripheral nerves are usually symmetrical, and roots are rarely symmetrical"***.
  The truth of this statement is apparent. However, I also mention that there are exceptions to this statement. In mononeuropathy multiplex, the peripheral nerves are asymmetrically involved initially and if untreated, will form a pattern of symmetrical distal polyneuropathy whereas in Guillain–Barré syndrome (GBS) the roots are usually mildly

asymmetrically involved. However, the statement ***"Peripheral Nerves tingle, Roots pain"*** remains true even for these exceptions.

- ***"Don't elicit reflexes, titrate them in this case"***.
  I make this statement when dealing with a case of reversible ischemic neurological deficit (RIND) or subtle hemiparesis. This statement has already been clarified in Chapters 12 and 14.
- ***"Subacute sclerosing pan encephalitis (SSPE) is always in the eyes"***.
  Over the years of observing patients with SSPE, it is my experience that the myoclonic jerks always begin in the eyes. Hence, in a patient with repeated myoclonic jerks of uncertain etiology, always look at the eyes at the beginning of the jerk. A bright resident doctor in Chennai heard this statement of mine, went back to the wards, and observed the myoclonic jerks of his patient. He ordered a second electroencephalogram (EEG) which was fairly classical for SSPE. Kindly note that early in SSPE, the EEG may not show characteristic repetitive discharges and at times several EEGs may be required.
- ***"Don't take one finding in isolation to make a diagnosis"***.
  Many postgraduates hinge their diagnosis from one prominent clinical finding. It is prudent to assess all the clinical findings, prominent or otherwise, before coming to any conclusion regarding the diagnosis. In my experience, this has happened particularly in the practical exams when I have been the examiner. They make a diagnosis based on a prominent clinical finding and tend to ignore all the other findings. Under such circumstances, I have found it very difficult to "unfix" the candidate from his/her diagnosis and guide them to the right path of clinical reasoning.
- ***"In a patient with diabetes and refractory giddiness, check the Romberg sign"***.
  I have already mentioned this point in Chapter 13.
- ***"A hot water bag and a paralyzed patient are never in the same bed"***.
  In the past, it was a common practice to give a hot water bag to a patient with paraplegia and urinary retention. Because of the sensory level, this only served to produce a burn injury on the lower abdomen. Fortunately, this is no longer practiced. Hot water bags or electric heating pads are still used as home remedies for pain, without realizing that it may be associated with a sensory loss. The patient, whom I described in Chapter 1, observation 2, had numbness over the left thigh (L2-3-4 lesion) and took hot water fomentations for his pain, only to burn himself over the left thigh. This statement must be emphasized to the lay public, general practitioners, and medical students at all levels of specialization.
- When palpating peripheral nerves in the limbs ***"Check the texture as well as the thickness of the nerve"***.
  This is not my statement but was made by Professor Darab K. Dastur, the renowned neuropathologist, who had done extensive work in leprosy. This statement of his is particularly true in the early part of leprous pathology or in a patient who has been treated for leprosy but has hidden the fact

because of the social stigma. In these two situations, the nerve may not be thickened but the texture is different. He further went on to explain to me that I should palpate the nerves with my fingertips and not the pulp of my fingers. The normal nerve is soft and rolls across your fingertips. The abnormal nerve is hard and "slips" under your fingertips. Only with practice will one be able to appreciate Dr Dastur's teaching.

Index

Page numbers followed by *b* refer to box, *f* refer to figure, *fc* refer to flowchart, and *t* refer to table.

D

E

N

O

P

Q

R

S

T

U

V

W

X

Z